COMPAÑEROS

LATINOS IN CHICAGO
AND THE MIDWEST

Series Editors
Frances R. Aparicio,
University of Illinois at Chicago
Pedro Cabán,
State University of New York
Juan Mora-Torres,
DePaul University
Maria de los Angeles Torres,
University of Illinois at Chicago

*A list of books in the series appears
at the end of this book.*

COMPAÑEROS

Latino Activists
in the Face of AIDS

JESUS RAMIREZ-VALLES

UNIVERSITY OF ILLINOIS PRESS

Urbana, Chicago, and Springfield

© 2011 by the Board of Trustees
of the University of Illinois
All rights reserved
Manufactured in the United States of America
1 2 3 4 5 C P 5 4 3 2 1
∞ This book is printed on acid-free paper.

Library of Congress Cataloging-in-Publication Data
Ramirez-Valles, Jesus.
Compañeros : Latino activists in the face of AIDS / Jesus Ramirez-Valles.
p. cm.
Includes bibliographical references and index.
ISBN 978-0-252-03644-6 (hbk. : alk. paper)
ISBN 978-0-252-07821-7 (pbk. : alk. paper)
1. Gay activists—United States. 2. AIDS activists—United States.
3. Hispanic American gays—Political activity—United States.
4. Hispanic American sexual minorities—Political activity—United States.
5. Gays—Identity. I. Title.
HQ76.8.U5R36   2011
362.196'9792008968073—dc23   2011027786

To my little Cameron

CONTENTS

Acknowledgments   ix

Introduction   1

Chapter 1.   Social-class Origins and Trajectories   19

Chapter 2.   Gender Deviants   37

Chapter 3.   The Meanings of Latino   63

Chapter 4.   The Formation of Gay and Trans Identities   81

Chapter 5.   Life with HIV and AIDS   100

Chapter 6.   Getting Involved   117

Chapter 7.   Finding Compañeros   138

Conclusion: The Road of Compañeros   156

Appendix   165

References   167

Index   175

ACKNOWLEDGMENTS

Gracias to all the participants who shared their life histories for this project. Their voices are the soul of this book. My heartfelt gratitude also goes to Rafael M. Díaz, who has inspired not only me but a generation of scholars. He was with me throughout this project giving me support, guidance, and a loving friendship. My friends from Juárez, Mexico, and El Paso, Texas, with whom I started organizing against AIDS, have been with me in this journey as well. They are my *compañeros*. Marco and Oscar, in particular, were my mentors. They showed me how to navigate life as a gay man. Our work shaped my views on AIDS, public health, and community.

I benefited from the terrific work of my research team: Dalia García, Raquel Vazquez, Lisa M. Kuhns, Jorge Sanchez, Antonio Jimenez, Andrea Heckert, Amanda Brown, Lilian Ferrer, Norberto Valbuena, and Dianna Manjarrez. They assisted me in various aspects of this project, from recruiting participants to interviewing, coding, and proofreading numerous versions of the manuscript. Their many contributions were vital to the success of the project.

A fellowship from the Center for AIDS Prevention Studies (CAPS) of the University of California at San Francisco helped me plant the seeds for this project. I want to especially acknowledge the mentorship and encouragement of Barbara Marin (then at CAPS) as well as the camaraderie of my fellow visiting professors at CAPS. I learned from all of you and you made my summers in San Francisco feel quite warm.

A grant from the National Institute of Mental Health (MH62937) provided me with generous financial resources. The late Louis Steinberg and Angela Pattatucci, from the National Institutes of Health, were key advocates of my work. I was also fortunate to receive a residency at the Bellagio Study Center from the Rockefeller Foundation. The stimulating intellectual discussions, friendship, and the idyllic beauty of Lake Como created an incomparable space to work. Especial credit to Pilar Palacia, director of the center, for making me feel at home and offering me her friendship. Likewise, a fellowship from the Great Cities Institute of the University of Illinois at Chicago and a Faculty Scholarship Support Award from the University of Illinois gave me the time and resources to prepare the manuscript for final submission.

This book served as an inspiration for my documentary film *Tal Como Somos/Just As We Are* (distributed by Films for the Humanities & Sciences at http://ffh.films.com). The film was superbly directed by Judith McCray and supported by a grant from the National Institute of Mental Health (R42 MH071157-02). I am indebted to the subjects in this film for their trust and their courage to share their lives in the big screen.

Frances Aparicio and Joan Mary Catapano opened the doors of the University of Illinois Press to this book. Thank you for believing in the value of *Compañeros*. I also genuinely appreciate the suggestions of the reviewers. Their candid and constructive comments helped me, I believe, better communicate my ideas.

I am grateful to Richard Rodriguez for his support and friendship. His comments and wisdom motivated me to revise sections of the book. After our lunch meeting in San Francisco, I ran to my hotel room and wrote the first five pages of the introduction. He helped me get closer to my own voice.

Finally, I want to say *muchas gracias* to my family and friends. There are no words to express adequately my gratitude to my mother and my father. They have always supported my dreams. My mother's hard work, particularly, allowed me to have the best education. Equally, I am grateful to my immediate family—my partner, Brad Trask, and our son, Cameron. I love you guys. You fill the daily little things of our life with joy.

If there is any good in this book, it is because of those who contributed to it. The shortcomings are mine alone.

INTRODUCTION

> Every story is, by definition, unfaithful. Reality . . . cannot
> be told or repeated. Reality can only be invented anew.
> —MARTÍNEZ 1995: 97

My first memories of AIDS are blurred. I do remember reading in *El Norte*, a Mexican national newspaper, something about homosexuals dying of a strange disease in the United States. It was a Sunday morning and I was in bed, in the two-room apartment I shared with a classmate. It was either 1985 or 1986 and I was in college, in Monterrey, Mexico. I did not know then that I was a gay man. I only knew I was different from most males and that I was attracted to men. Nor did I know how such a disease, AIDS, would shape my life.

A few years later, in my hometown of Ciudad Juárez, on the Mexico–United States border, I was organizing with other gay men and sex workers to address HIV/AIDS prevention and treatment. I was living at my mother's home and had developed a circle of gay friends. In Juárez and neighboring El Paso, Texas, I met Marco, Oscar, and José. They were gay men, older than I, who taught me what it was like to be a gay man. We were, and still remain, very close friends. The four of us began the first organized efforts to fight the epidemic among gay men in Juárez, Mexico. My three *compañeros* (see the *Compañeros* section later in this introduction for an explanation of this term), and others with whom we would meet, put me on the road to adulthood, on a career path, and on a journey to write this book about the lives of *compañeros*.

After college, I returned to Juárez, where I found a job with a national women's organization, working on reproductive health and economic development issues in Mexico. In this organization, I was first exposed to grassroots public health. The organization's base was made up of women who were leaders in their *colonias* (neighborhoods) and workplaces. The organization had started an HIV/AIDS prevention program with sex workers, both females and transvestites. Juárez had a well-earned reputation as a prostitution and drinking town. The *maquiladoras* (assembly plants) and the military base in El Paso sustained its economy, which was made up mainly of bars, cantinas, drug traffic, and prostitution. The distinction persists, as shown in the 2005 gay cowboy film *Brokeback Mountain*. Ang Lee, the director, sends one of the main characters, a good-looking white gay man, across the border to Juárez in search of sex. There he walks into the narrow dark streets of the red-light district, where brown women and men offer their bodies.

I became involved in the organization's prevention program with women and transvestite sex workers in 1988. HIV and AIDS became salient in my life, professionally and personally. Then, one night over drinks in the gay bar that we visited almost every weekend, Marco, Oscar, and I decided to work together to address HIV and AIDS in the gay community. We would combine our talents and our free time. Marco was a handsome and charismatic engineer. Oscar was a physician and a teacher, while I was an organizer and an educator with access to a public health organization. We began by organizing talks at men's homes during the weekends. With the help of José, who worked in a relatively wealthy AIDS organization in El Paso, we arranged access to HIV testing and some medications.

We soon found ourselves at the center of a much larger group of men, organizing hundreds of other gay men, meeting and recruiting men in the cruising parks and streets, distributing condoms, and conducting fund-raising events in discos and bars. We got some funding through our association with the women's organization I worked for, which had received a grant from a U.S. foundation. The media referred to us as "the leaders of the gay community." We also found ourselves taking care of those *compañeros* dying of AIDS. The images of those we cared for and of those we buried are the most vivid memories I have of that time in my life. Twenty-five years later, the faces of our *compañeros*, their bodies lying in hospital beds, and their funeral services still haunt me.

But my times in Juárez and El Paso with Marco, Oscar, José, and the other *compañeros* were not all about illness, death, and hardships. While we took our community work very seriously, we enjoyed it fully, or at least I did. The work became part of our own lives as it took over our evenings and weekends. It became part of our friendship and our gayness. The camaraderie even among strangers, filled our souls, gave us energy to do more than we were doing already, and ignited our creativity.

Oscar used to say that each gay man's death represented a missing book in the library. The death of a young gay man represented a book that was never written or completed. The analogy is not original, but it resonated in me because of my own love for books and because my grandfather did not get to complete his own book. In the later years of his life, my grandfather's dream was to write a book. His was an engineering textbook. He dedicated many hours of his day to writing, by hand, in a little notebook. Years after his death, I still look at his notebook and the small book collection he left behind in my mother's home.

This book, *Compañeros*, tells the story of contemporary Latino gay and bisexual men and transgender individuals (GBTs), who, like many of my friends, joined the fight against AIDS. In *Compañeros* I describe their trajectories as activists and the processes by which they have forged a space for themselves in light of their marginalization. All the contributing activists are of Latin American origin or descent and live in the United States. I met them and collected their life histories more than a decade after my own initiation in the AIDS movement and my relocation to the United States.

When we started that work in Juárez, we did not know we were part of a large international and transnational phenomenon called the AIDS movement. Nor did we see ourselves as activists or volunteers. We were just doing what we thought we were supposed to do. We were doing what came out naturally from our individual and collective energies. Only later did we learn that our small efforts reflected larger-scale endeavors in places such as San Francisco, New York City, Chicago, Mexico City, Guadalajara, London, and Rio de Janeiro.

Our work, however, was different from what was taking place in the north, especially New York and San Francisco, and across the ocean, in London and Paris. We did not have the financial resources needed to launch large prevention and treatment programs. Even now, medical therapies to fight HIV are not widely available in Mexico. Also, our collective efforts were not embedded in identity politics, which dominated the social landscape in the United States. We were not defined as "gay men" or "queer people" fighting AIDS. Nor were we white, Latino, or black men. We were a group of men (albeit, marginalized) organized around AIDS. Of course, within the group and among the men we worked with, it was assumed that we were homosexuals or gay. Even with some of the *compañeros*, we were "amigas." In dealing with the outside world, we refused to use a label. In the views of outsiders, we were just a bunch of homosexual men, with all the marginalization and stigma it implied at that time in Mexico.

None of us wanted to be publicly labeled as gay, homosexual, or *joto* (derogatory, faggot). Our families, including my own, had some knowledge of our homosexuality. Most of us also lived with our parents and siblings, which is still the custom for unmarried adults south of the Rio Bravo. Family members knew we hung out mostly with other men and some even met our boyfriends (but without identifying them as such). Our private lives, which included male friends, weekend gatherings at the bars, and boyfriends, were never explicitly discussed.

Our counterparts north of the border might have said that we were "in the closet," but that would be an easy answer—not to mention arrogant. To say that our realities, as Mexican homosexual men, were and, to some extent, still are more complex than those of white gay men in the United States would also be an easy answer. We were navigating through different social spaces that were at times contradictory but not completely separated. These included our family lives, our Catholicism, our childhood friends, our homosexual friends, our lovers, our coworkers, and our work in combating AIDS. We were trying to prevent any possible rupture or crash. The realities of us, *compañeros,* were not made up of identities based on sexual desire, "lifestyle," or skin color. That was the case in our own little corner of Mexico (and in the backyard of the United States), anyway. In other parts of the country, such as Mexico City and Guadalajara, there were people marching on the streets claiming "orgullo homosexual" (gay pride). That was not our world.

Our strategy in fighting HIV/AIDS was also different from the one deployed by groups in the north, particularly the AIDS Coalition to Unleash Power (ACT UP), which led the AIDS movement in the United States and some European countries. ACT UP employed what is called direct action (Fisher 2005; Shaw 1996). The strategy is a form of social protest aimed at making direct demands on those believed to have the power to change an unjust situation. The actions of ACT UP included disrupting international AIDS conferences, "storming" the National Institutes of Health, and interfering with church services inside St. Patrick's Roman Catholic Cathedral in New York City. The membership of ACT UP reflected that of the AIDS movement in the late 1980s and early 1990s: mostly white gay men. The organization succeeded in changing the course of the epidemic by making the state responsive to the devastation taking place in gay communities (Chambré 2006; Epstein 1996; Kobasa 1990).

We were doing none of that. We did not call ourselves gay men. Moreover, Mexico did not, and does not, have the resources to respond to the epidemic, even if we had demanded access to treatment. In the face of such a reality, we did not have the sense of entitlement so common among gays in the United States. Our strategy could be defined as underground community development. It was underground because we operated in a homosexual culture within spaces outside of the public view, in private homes, at night, and in clandestine bars and bathhouses. We did not want to reveal ourselves to the larger public because the public censure that would inevitably result would have prevented many men from working with us. Indeed, most of the men we worked with did not use a gay identity in public. We worked with physicians, nurses, and Roman Catholic priests. We made some demands of them, but we did not confront them. We got others, such as hospitals and priests, to work with us through our social networks. A colleague of mine, for instance, had a friend who was a Jesuit priest. Through her, we would arrange for a priest to conduct Masses for our dead *compañeros*.

While working with the women's organization and with the men in the fight against AIDS, I met professionals and academics from the United States who had degrees in public health. They would come on behalf of the funders to evaluate or train us. They opened the doors of a public health career in the United States for me. When I was about to finish college and return to Ciudad Juárez, I knew I wanted to pursue a research or academic career in mass communications. Public health did not yet exist as an option for me. I also knew I did not want to stay on the border.

Growing up, I was one of the few Mexicans I knew who did not dream of living in the United States. I grew up in a large working-class family. We had some very rough times. Somehow, I developed an antigringo and anticapitalist outlook, which was not uncommon in the Americas of the 1960s and 1970s. In high school I was fascinated by Marx and Engels and angered by the U.S. invasion of Nicaragua and Chile.

So, despite living on the border (or because of it), I did not dream of a life in the United States. But I enjoyed what I knew about public health. I moved to Michigan to study public health, leaving my friends and *compañeros*. I also left AIDS behind, temporarily.

When I resumed my work on HIV/AIDS, this time in Chicago in the late 1990s, things had changed. The AIDS movement in the late 1990s and early 2000s had ceased to be grassroots efforts that produced direct action. It had become the "AIDS industry" (Patton 1989). Many of us who had once provided services and mobilized people in the streets and our homes with little in the way of financial resources, had become health professionals, administrators, and academics. Now, white middle-class gay men, dressed in tuxedos and posing for the press, put their talents into fund-raising social events. The movement became an industry and part of the system, as it gained access to resources particularly at the federal level. It likewise found its impetus in the ability of medical treatments to help curb death rates. The fight shifted. It was once between grassroots groups and the state. Now, it is among social service organizations. Sean Strub, the founder of *Poz* magazine, rightly noted: "AIDS had become a huge industry that has made careers, fame and fortune for many. But the rush over the corpses and voices of people with HIV in the pursuit of power, institutionalization and fundraising has been disgraceful" (Strub 2005).

As the AIDS movement lost its force and became mainstream, the gay movement followed suit. The radical and critical stance that the gay movement brought in the 1960s and 1970s faded away as the fear of AIDS increased. Stigmatization increased. Activists and volunteers joined the non-profit and public sectors. The stance against marriage and the hierarchical family structure quickly shifted, as did the pride of being different and the principles of loving each other and expressing our sexual beings free of social, religious, and legal constraints. The gay movement exchanged those notions for a right to marry, monogamy, safe sex, and inclusion.

That is the melancholia that Douglas Crimp (2002) talks about, borrowing from Freud. The violence of the AIDS epidemic made some of us vanish in fear and denial. Others had no other option but to confront it. They are the ones who endured the fight, the deaths, the medications, and the ignominy. As Crimp points out, such a violent force eventually took over. Gay men (and their allies) were emptied; they were physically and emotionally exhausted. Their sense of themselves was shattered. Melancholy set in, creating a fertile soil for conservatism to breed.

Yet, in the midst of this melancholia, I began to hear personal stories of transformation—perhaps as a sign of things to come. Gay men were speaking openly about how AIDS transformed their lives and inspired their activism. These stories of personal triumph contrasted with the larger story—the decline of the AIDS and gay movement. This was unlike what I witnessed in Mexico and became the seed of *Compañeros*. I became interested in exploring gay and transgender people's efforts to overcome the threat of death and the possibility of change that the closeness of death brings.

I wanted to study and document stories of GBT activists in the AIDS movement in the United States, especially the accounts of those of Latin American origin or descent. Scholars and the general media have overlooked the work and the voices of Latino GBTs in the AIDS movement creating a void in the history of the AIDS (and gay) movement, the social sciences, and public health in the United States. This is troubling because ethnic and sexual minorities are currently more affected by the epidemic than their white counterparts (Catania et al. 2001; Wolitski et al. 2001), and because the larger Latino population in the United States is less supportive of civil liberties for homosexuals than for whites and African Americans. Nationally, 72 percent of Latinos feel that sex between two adults of the same sex is unacceptable compared to 59 percent of whites (Pew Hispanic Center/Kaiser Family Foundation 2003). The absence of Latino GBTs' voices hinders our understanding of how a group already marginalized because of their ethnicity and skin color confronts adversity, such as the AIDS epidemic. How do they get involved in the AIDS movement? How do they confront the racial discrimination in a white-dominated movement? How do they handle their family and culture's beliefs about AIDS and homosexuality? Without their accounts, thus, the history of the AIDS movement remains incomplete.

The idea for this book began to materialize one sunny afternoon on a beach in Puerto Rico, where I was attending a conference. I was with Rafael, a new *compañero* and mentor I had met in the United States. He was a professor in San Francisco; I was living in Chicago, beginning my professorial career. I shared with him my thoughts about the transformation stories of activists. He believed in the idea and suggested that I also look at the role of activism in overcoming homophobia and racism. I have walked one full circle: our conversation and his idea took me back to my times on the border.

Compañeros is about the lives of eighty Latino activists and volunteers. Seventy-two identify themselves as gay men, three as bisexual, and five as transgender (male to female). All of them have been involved in the AIDS movement either in the United States, in Latin America, or in both. They have participated in either AIDS or lesbian, gay, bisexual, and transgender (LGBT) organizations fighting HIV and AIDS. I chronicle their lives, from childhood to the present, as told by them in an effort to understand how people become activists and the role of activism in their lives. I also look at their subjective experience as ethnic and sexual minorities and how they intersect with their involvement in AIDS organizations. The names of all activists and volunteers interviewed for this study are fictional to protect their identities.

Activism and the Self

A central thesis of *Compañeros* is that community involvement, such as activism and volunteerism, while creating social change, also nourishes and transforms the self. As a particular form of social participation, it is about the self as much as it is about working for one's community and society (Bellah et al. 1996). Researchers of the AIDS movement have shown that participation fosters self-esteem and social support (Bebbington and Gatter 1994; Boehmer 2000; Chambré 1991; Kobasa 1990, 1991; Omoto and Crain 1995; Snyder and Omoto 1992). Orlando, one activist in this book, notes that many white, brown, and black gay men came to call themselves "warriors" through their participation. They were victims—not of a virus, but of a social system that fears sexual expression and difference. But they refused to go quietly.

The premise that activism and volunteerism are vital to the development of the self and to the creation of an identity comes from the French sociologist Émile Durkheim (1951). In this theory of social integration (S. Cohen 1988; House 1981; Pearlin et al. 1981) he offers that participation through volunteerism and activism links individuals to the larger society and provides them with social support and a sense of themselves. Participation also enables individuals to deal with stressors, such as racial discrimination and homophobia (Meyer 1995; Williams et al. 2003; Ensel and Lin 1991). In some instances, however, those means of participation may become stressors, as when individuals experience burnout or conflicts within the group.

Community involvement enhances self-worth because it provides interaction with peers (Ramirez-Valles 2002; Allahyari 2000; Frable et al. 1997). This is particularly relevant for those who do not conform to dominant gender roles and identities, because their peers are not readily available. Peers, like *compañeros*, give us a point of reference about who we are, as well as feedback and guidance. In addition, both volunteerism and activism create an identity of being a caring and good person, and a competent and active citizen (Kobasa 1990; Moen and Fields 1999; Turner et al. 1993; Youniss and Yates 1997). My colleagues and I have found that Latino GBTs who are involved in AIDS organizations have access to social networks and face-to-face interactions, and cultivate a sense of community (Ramirez-Valles and Díaz 2005; Ramirez-Valles and Brown 2003; Ramirez-Valles 2002).

These features of activism are especially significant when we consider the stigma that GBTs, and Latinos in particular, endure. Stigma based on gender nonconformity, skin color, or HIV and AIDS creates undue stress because it places demands on individuals, exceeding their resources or abilities to respond. GBTs within Latino communities experience what Cathy Cohen (1999) refers to as "secondary marginalization." They, as a group, are excluded and silenced by the larger Latino communities. Through activism, GBTs, including Latinos, cope with, offset, or buffer the damage caused by such stigma (Weitz 1991; Ramirez-Valles et al. 2005).

Compañeros

At the heart of being involved, and at the center of these life histories, is the idea of finding the self in the company of others. Activists and volunteers join movements, grassroots organizations, and social service organizations for multiple reasons, ranging from creating a just world to helping the sick (Musick and Wilson 2008). In doing so, they find out who they are. They create an identity and a place in the world. But this sense of self does not refer solely to the "who I am," such as a gay man, a Latino man, a transgender person, or a person living with AIDS. It includes core values about what is good and just, relationships with others and the wider society, and citizenship. Perhaps most importantly, it comprises the ability to create and live a fulfilling life. In the particular instance of Latino GBTs, community involvement means finding the means to live, survive, and create a self at the margin of society. It is about creating life in the margin, while trying to expand, shrink, or remove that same margin.

In getting involved in the AIDS movement, I propose, activists and volunteers find *compañeros,* with whom they construct individual and collective identities. The word itself, *compañeros,* encompasses a quality in our relationships with others that is not conveyed by any single word in the English language. I first heard and used this word in the AIDS context, when I was working with a women's organization in Mexico. The colleague who was coordinating the HIV prevention program with women and transvestite sex workers used it regularly in reference to the people with whom she worked. She would say "*las compañeras* this" and "*las compañeras* that." It was her way of establishing a not-so-hierarchical relationship with the sex workers (who obviously were different from her and had far fewer resources than she) and among the sex workers themselves. She also used it to convey the democratic and collaborative process characteristic of her work with those women and transvestites. Marco, Oscar, José, and I would also refer to *compañeros* when working with the gay men.

I heard the term *compañeros* again in Santiago de Chile, during a visit in the early 2000s. I visited two organizations working on AIDS, which then were the sole bases of the incipient AIDS movement in Chile. I felt as if I had traveled, not only in space but also in time, back to the late 1980s and early 1990s in Ciudad Juárez. The *colonias,* the brown expressive faces, the welcoming hugs, the animated conversations over cigarettes and coffee, the ever-expanding time, the anger for the government's refusal to act, and the idealism and hope made me feel at home with the Chilean *compañeros* fighting AIDS. The men and the women in both organizations also used the terms *compañeros* and *compañeras* when referring to members of the organization and to their constituencies.

The word *compañero* entails a relationship of solidarity among equals. In the context of the social movement, it means walking a road together. This relationship is not based on a balance of exchanges, as are relationships in the United States. It is based on a felt commitment and obligation. The relationship is not contractual, compartmentalized, and shallow like those relationships that we create (and detest) in white and gay communities in the United States. This relationship is profound, heartfelt, and complete. It is what Deborah Gould calls in *Moving Politics* (2009) an "affective state." This sense of *compañero* is far from that uttered by Fidel Castro in his Communist rhetoric. It is very close to the experiences of many of these Latino GBT activists. It authentically echoes their own voices.

In making the claim that community involvement is about creating the self and finding *compañeros,* I am drawing partially from Robert Bellah and his colleagues' *Habits of the Heart* (Bellah et al. 1996), one of the most influential works on American culture and community involvement of the twentieth century. Following Alexis de Tocqueville's tradition (1830/2000), Bellah and his colleagues propose that a distinctive feature of American culture is the notion of getting involved. Volunteering, activism, and membership in organizations are vital to the individuals' connection to their society and the maintenance of the so-called democratic institutions. This notion is at the center of American culture (Putnam 2000). It is therefore a constant concern among social scientists and practitioners in the helping professions, because the individual precedes and, in many instances, supersedes the collective in white middle-class America. The concern, then, becomes finding a balance between the "I" and the "We."

Even when an individual joins and creates connection with others and a sense of self, he or she does it in a utilitarian and individualistic manner. The individual uses the involvement to connect with others and find a sense of self, but the sense of self comes from within. The individual chooses what to take from others, and how, when, and where to get involved.

In the context of the U.S. mainstream culture, there is a clear distinction between the individual and the group or collectivity, and between paid and unpaid work. The terms *activist* and *volunteer,* hence, serve to define ways by which individuals can connect to the group and to society. They refer to ways in which individuals can participate in the wider society, other than as a worker, mother, son, or elected official. Those terms are also part of a vocabulary that defines and separates social spheres, such as work, family, church, politics, and leisure typical of the compartmentalized society in the United States. In many Latin American contexts, the distinctions between the "I" and "We," or between the individual and the collective, and among different social spheres are generally vague and of less significance than in the United States. Thus, actions such as helping others, social disobedience, marches, and struggles for fair housing take place through relationships of solidarity, mutual help, extended families, political parties, and unions. There is no language, or role, to restore the connection between the individual and society. The individual is in the collective.

Thus, the premises of community involvement among white Americans and among Latinos and Latin Americans differ: The separation between the "I" and the "We," the self and the collective, is blurred and of minor significance in the latter. In addition, the "utilitarian individualism" and "expressive individualism" that typify U.S. culture (Bellah et al. 1996), are absent in (if not antithetical to) the Latino cultural context. As a result, it is difficult to find *compañeros* among white Americans. There are no *compañeros* to walk the road with and create a sense of self. The *compañeros* are Latinos.

I do not mean to suggest that Latino and white GBTs are essentially different from one another or that Latinos (or whites) are a monolithic group. The life histories of these activists actually show important variations in the identities and experiences of Latino GBTs. Likewise, the history of ACT UP illustrates exceptional instances in which ties of solidarity are created across different groups in the United Sates (Chambré 2006; Gould 2009; Stockdill 2003). I argue that there are differences in cultural and social patterns of relating. These patterns are general and, while dominant, are not universally displayed by every single individual. Thus, they may not apply to every individual's behaviors and beliefs.

Latinoness

The Latino experience as represented in the life histories of these men and transgender activists is distinctive in other ways. The uniqueness, however, does not rest on essentialist ideas of race and ethnicity. The essentialist (and racist) discourse states that so-called Latinos are inherently different from and inferior to "whites." It further posits that those differences emerge from our distinct physiology and genetic composition. As if this notion needed a logical and scientific rebuttal, social scientists, historians, and geneticists have provided evidence that physiology and genes do not determine character and that the genetic variation is greater within racial groups than across them (Wilkinson and King 1987; Cooper and David 1986). Skin color, language, and place of birth are meaningless, unless we make them meaningful. They are relevant only to the extent that they affect our life chances, the places we live, the schools we attend, the jobs we perform, and the income we earn.

Immigration is one aspect that most defines the Latino experience. The separation and subsequent fracture when one leaves home mark the new life in the United States. Such a mark persists through generations. Its significance is diminished as generations pass. Latinoness vanishes as generations of immigrants settle in the United States and lessen contact with Latin America. Half of the activists in *Compañeros* are immigrants, while the other half are descended from immigrants. Unlike me, most immigrants came to the United States to make a living. Many of them grew up with very limited financial resources in Latin America. They and their parents came to look for better opportunities, which effort netted them only low-paying jobs at the bottom of the labor market.

Immigration also creates a conflict between yearning for home and being unwilling or unable to go back and re-create a life there. Home is family, friends, *compañeros*, laughter, amorphous time, warmhearted relationships, and lively conversations over meals. Home is where we are not identified as brown. Yet, the home we miss once suffocated and betrayed us. The home in which we once lived is now physically distant. It could not provide, nor allow, different selves to be realized. It could not let free spirits wander. Nor could it give us the freedom that money and anonymity offer in the United States.

For some *compañeros* in this book, being the sons and daughters of immigrants means not being able to fully join either the white American culture or the brown Latin American culture. They feel a part of those two worlds, but both worlds reject them. They resent being abandoned. The Latino with broken Spanish and flawless English does not have access to Latin America, because he or she does not have the language (*lingua mater*) with which to create and reproduce culture. He, or she, only has English, which does not create but alienates Latin Americans. Neither does this Latino have access to America, because America rejects his brown skin and his yearning for the home that his parents talk about.

In the stories of these *compañeros* we also find two predominant figures—family and mother. The family (nuclear and extended) is where we first derive our identities as sons, daughters, brothers, and sisters. The family is our connection to the outside world—or to other families, the state, the larger society, the labor market, and to God. I left my family home after high school, but this is an exception. Most of us do not leave our families to go and create "families of choice." We remain obligated to the families of our childhood. Yet, for those who do not conform to the dominant gender roles, the importance of family generates great tension. It is, at once, a supportive and oppressive force. After all, the family is still the basis of our gendered system. There is little room for being gay or transgender.

The other figure, mother, has been a constant presence in our collective imagery. She appears in Octavio Paz's Malinche, the Virgin of Guadalupe, Eva Perón, María Félix, and in Pedro Almodóvar's melodramas. According to the archetype, mother is a stoic protector, provider, accomplice, supporter, and a victim of the patriarchal man—our father. A mother is in charge of the house. She must make home look harmonious even when it is not. This archetype takes a tragic quality in the son's imagery. Mother and daughter can freely be equals, friends, rivals, or accomplices. A son is tragically connected to the mother in pain, betrayal, abandonment, or joy. A son, the gay and the transgender son, is subjugated by the mother.

Uniqueness aside, there is a universal property in the life histories of these GBTs. There are themes that they share with other activists and with other GBTs across the Americas. They live in the margin created by a gender and racial system, a religious (Catholic) ideology, and by an epidemic. While pushed to the margin, they create life and culture there, and they fight against those forces that sustain their marginality. Like other men who do not conform to the dominant gender identities and roles, they must find ways to create a space to be and to function in their societies. Still, I must note that some want to stay on the periphery, for that is where they find comfort, freedom, and the richness of life. They do not want to be part of the society's core. The universality, then, lies in the oppression, in the pain, and in the deprivation that oppression brings. It also lies in the resiliency and the struggle caused, unintentionally, by that oppression. Last, it lies in the constant search for a sense of oneself.

Making Life Histories

Compañeros is made up of life histories. A life history is a fairly complete account of one's entire life experience, in which one presents the self to others highlighting major aspects of the self and one's life (Atkinson 1998). The life history typically follows a sequence of events on a time line. It contains events or characters related by a structure. Although it can be thought of as a narrative, it compromises several (smaller) narratives or stories (Maines 1993). The life history of a Latino gay man, for example, may include a story about how he became an activist, a story about becoming gay, and a story about his education.

Storytelling is pervasive in our everyday lives (Denzin 1989; Riessman 1993). It is hard to think of our actions and our own selves outside of stories. The stories that we tell and our life histories communicate more than discrete "facts" about life. They constitute our subjective experience, our lived and interpreted experience (Ewick and Selby 1995; Gergen 1988; Cortazzi 1993; Hydén 1997). But they are not an individual creation. They are the product of the social group in which they are located and rendered meaningful. We tell stories about ourselves drawing from the vocabularies and conventions available in our social groups. In this sense, a life history does not represent a true or an authentic self; rather, it represents a social self (Somers 1992).

I tell the story of these activists through their own woven stories because their voices best represent who they are and how they have come to be activists. Their life histories illustrate the richness of the cultures and the social milieu in which they live. In their life histories, their childhood, families, friends, boyfriends, and *compañeros* come alive. We witness the schools and churches that they attended, and the ones to which they now belong. We see the state and its public health institutions, and how a viral infection exposes their flaws by creating a social epidemic. Also, we learn about the groups that these activists have created and the struggles upon which they have embarked. It is through their life histories that we can see how they become brown, gay, transgender, HIV positive, people living with AIDS, and activists. Furthermore, the life histories offer us a window to the progression of the AIDS movement.

I collected these life histories between 2001 and 2002, with the assistance of a staff of five bilingual interviewers in Chicago and San Francisco (see the appendix for the demographic information of the participants; data are separated by city only for informative purposes). I chose these two cities to capture a large variety of Latino GBTs and because of my familiarity with them, not to make a comparative analysis. In both cities, the majority of Latin Americans are of Mexican origin, but in San Francisco we find more GBT immigrants from other Latin American countries than are found in Chicago. For many gay men in Latin America, San Francisco epitomizes gay life; hence, they immigrate there. Moreover, the latter has been the epicenter of the AIDS epidemic. This means that the prevalence of HIV/AIDS is higher and that Latino GBTs are more likely to get involved in AIDS and LGBT affairs in San Francisco than in Chicago.

The recruitment strategy aimed at making careful generalizations about the lives of Latino GBT participants in the AIDS movement in major urban centers in the United States. The main enrollment criteria was to have been involved, as activist or volunteer, in HIV/AIDS issues at any point in their lifetime. Then, I aimed at creating a diverse sample by seeking participation from different subgroups defined by HIV status, country of origin (e.g., United States, Puerto Rico, Mexico), and main language spoken. These variables shape the lives of Latino GBTs and, hence, the manner in which they engage in the AIDS movement. For example, the experience of race is qualitatively different between those born and raised in the United States and those raised in Latin America. Likewise, being HIV positive propels, in many instances, community involvement to fight AIDS, whereas those who are HIV negative have a different route to activism. Nonetheless, we know very little about Latino GBTs as to speak with certainty about which (and how) factors influence their lives, especially in the times of AIDS. It is the purpose of this book to contribute to such knowledge.

The interviewers and I recruited and met these GBTs through community-based organizations, newspaper ads, and through their own referrals. We sat with them, and with an audiotape recorder between us, asked them to tell us about their lives, from their first memories to the present. Then, I analyzed the interviews as a group, paying attention to the themes that developed organically within them. I focused on what was salient and rich in their life histories. I chose not to analyze and present their lives individually, because I would have not been able to put them in a dialogue with each other and underscore their collective nature. Instead, I knitted them together to create a single story (with some deviations). Thus, the reader will meet and get to know these *compañeros* through narratives of different aspects of their lives placed in thematically organized chapters.

The book is organized by themes and follows, to the extent possible, the structure of life histories. I first introduce these activists with a description of the social class positions in which they grew up and the ones they currently occupy. In chapter 2 I describe the stigmatization that these activists have encountered, from childhood to the present, because of their gender nonconformity. Here I also discuss the ways in which these activists confront such stigmatization. I follow this with the subject of race (chapter 3). I analyze the stigmatization that these activists have endured because they are defined as a racial group, different from the white majority. I also present the various and contradictory meanings of "Latino" among this group, and the ways in which the idea of race and the meanings of Latino become part of these individuals' activism and worldview.

In chapter 4 I focus on these activists' stories of becoming gay or transgender, from the moment they first felt different from others, to the point when they publicly assume those identities and use them to get community involved. Next, I turn to the experiences of those activists who are HIV positive or living with AIDS (chapter 5). Here I include accounts of becoming HIV positive, the impact on their lives and their loved ones, as well as the mechanisms for coping and confronting the illness. Finally, in chapters 6 and 7, I discuss how these activists became involved in the AIDS movement and the changes that involvement has brought to their lives.

In the concluding chapter I address what the lives of these Latino GBTs tell us about the current state of the AIDS and gay movements in the United States. I also take up the present and future state of Latinos (and Latinoness) and its presence in the United States queer landscape.

As I wrote the stories of these *compañeros,* I found comfort, hope, and lessons in life. I did not experience this when I was conversing with them with a tape recorder between us, and my interview script at my side, on my lap, or in my head. I relish the time I had with all these activists during the interviews. I did not know many of these men and transgenders before we met for our interview. I knew only a few of them. And I remain in contact only with a small number. I connected with most of them as a brown, gay man, immigrant, and as Mexican. I found in them aspects of life I have missed and yearned for. I cried with Bernardo when he was telling me about the love he had for his grandfather and the sadness after his death. I laughed with Vladimir's crafty, poetic, and cheerful use of Spanish. I enjoyed Blanca's deep voice serenading me with "Cucu-rru-cucu Paloma." I reminisced about my days in Cuba with Pierre (he was barefoot during the interview because of the torrential rains falling that morning; he entered my office all soaked and took his shoes and socks off). With Carmelo, I wondered how our paths had crossed, again, as we both grew up and witnessed the rise of AIDS on the border. We even had friends in common. And with Fabian, I traced the houses I had lived in Monterrey when I was a student. We had lived in the same neighborhood, when we were both students. But we were in different colleges, so we never met.

As I was writing them, these stories came alive to me. I became close to these *compañeros* as I typed and cobbled their stories together. Their stories became real and part of me. The writing made me think about them. I internalized them and understood them in a way that a conversation did not allow me to. Writing about them opened up spaces of my own life, some of which I had ignored (or closed off) for most of my adult life.

I found comfort in seeing in others pieces of the life I have lived, with the same pains, dreams, joys, and sins. The same comfort many of these *compañeros* have found through their lives in joining AIDS, Latino, and LGBT organizations. I felt comfort in learning that some of them also had days when there was nothing but beans and tortillas to eat. We became kindred spirits when I learned that they felt different when they went to a middle-class school, or when they were around other boys. They, like me, love their mothers, fathers, and siblings, but they want to and must be apart from them.

I found hope and peace in being reminded that in life there is pain, but also joy. There is life in oppression and in illness. While social forces might put us in the margin of society and life, there is pleasure, creativity, and energy to be found on the edge. Life might be fuller and richer in the margin, with *compañeros*.

Despite (or with) the forces of the state, church, gender, and epidemics, I found that people survive and have a sense of fullness in their lives (even if frequently ephemeral). They find joy and a sense of themselves in their families, lovers, partners, *compañeros,* and in working to change those forces. At times, I felt as if destiny, or a larger godlike force, had put these *compañeros* in front of me to see my own self, my soul, in order to prepare me for the life to come. In these last few years, I have lived with these stories. I have grown older. I have experienced new aspects of life. The changes I have undergone have been less painful and less startling because these *compañeros* prepared me. They warned me through their stories.

I trust that you, the reader, will find in these stories not only the consequences of the violent and arrogant forces of power and nature, but also hope, comfort, peace, and the lessons that life has to offer. You will find, like I did, the energy and the creativity that comes from living in the margins.

CHAPTER ONE

SOCIAL-CLASS ORIGINS
AND TRAJECTORIES

Social-class origins determine our life chances (McDonough and Berglund 2003; Feinstein 1993). It shapes our education, occupation, health status, migration, and life style. Latino GBTs who experience poverty also experience low levels of self-esteem and social support, and high levels of HIV and sexual risk behaviors (Díaz and Ayala 2001; Ramirez-Valles and Díaz 2005).

I grew up in something between a poor and a working-class family. At times we had nothing to eat but beans and potatoes. But my mother supported our education; she never asked us, or pushed us, to work or to leave school for a job. My mother raised us pretty much on her own, with sporadic financial support from my father and my grandfather. We were six siblings, five bothers and one sister.

I remained keenly aware of the social-class structures around me as I finished college and slowly climbed up to middle-class status. The women's health organization I was working for was run by a wealthy woman. The board of directors was made up of members of the elite families of Ciudad Juárez. The staff was a mix of middle-class professionals and working-class professionals, such as social workers and accountants. The people we were working for were very poor. They lived in the poorest areas of Mexico; in the outskirts of metropolitan areas, mostly.

There, I began to feel uncomfortable with my social-class position and that of the people we worked for. Although I developed good relationships with some of them, I did not like revealing my social-class status. Many times, I felt we were using them. I thought that I could not do anything to change the world they lived in; that my job held little meaning, if any, for them. I would feel "middle-class guilt," while detesting the charitable attitude of the middle class. This guilt was about the contrasts between classes; between what I had and what they did not have. To this date, I'm still conflicted.

With Marco, Oscar, José, and the other *compañeros* it was a little different. Our work against AIDS was not based on job relationships or on a professional-client relationship. We came and worked together as friends and *compañeros*. Our class differences were not significant and, even if they were, I did not see them as an obstacle. I did not feel as conflicted as I had with the women in the women's health organization. I was aware of the differences between most of the guys and me, especially in terms of education and income. I felt connected with them, while conscious that I was different from most of them; our life paths perhaps would not have crossed if it were not for AIDS.

My purpose in this chapter is to present examples in the form of vignettes of the social-class origins of these *compañeros*. Although I cannot establish any causal connection between the social class in which they were born and the events in their youth or adulthood, I propose that social-class origins did shape some of their life circumstances. That is, the social-class location of the families in which the activists were raised was one factor, if not the most significant, among several, shaping their life courses. For instance, some of the men who grew up in a poor or working-class environment began working early in their childhood or youth, did not go to college, and emigrated (either with their families or by themselves) to the United States. As adults, some of them also experienced homelessness and unemployment. Only in very few instances are these Latino GBTs able to change the course set by the social class into which they were born. The improvement some of them have made in their social-class standing, however, has been due to their own resiliency or to random events.

I see social class as an individual's location in the relations of production (Wright et al. 1982; Liberatos et al. 1988). There are three productive assets that largely determine social-class position: the actual means of production (e.g., capital, technology), authority within organizational structures, and credentials—for example, education and skills (Wright et al. 1982). Analytically, it is difficult to separate social class from factors such as race and migration. In the United States, in particular, social class and race are frequently connected. In the stories of Latino GBTs who were born or raised here, descriptions of the families' financial situation and the parents' occupation often overlap with references to race. As social-class theorists have argued (Roediger 1991; Wolpe 1986; Anthias 1990), social class and race are intertwined, affecting life circumstances, place of residency, schooling, peers, and occupational options. This intersection of social class and race (or, specifically, skin color) is not absent in the stories of those men born and raised in Latin American countries. The frequency and intensity of this intersection, however, is lower than among those born or raised in the United States.

I assessed social-class origins by two means. First, I made a categorization based on activists' own evaluation of their families' financial situation when they were growing up. Second, I assigned a social class based on several indicators, such as parents' occupation, home ownership, automobile ownership, and private or public elementary school attendance. This analysis resulted in the distributions shown in table 1. In addition, table 1 includes the social-class distribution in adulthood. The latter was assessed as the social-class standing at the time of the interview. I based this on similar factors, such as formal education, employment, home ownership, car ownership, and individuals' own appraisals.

There are no meaningful differences between social-class origins of the activists in Chicago and San Francisco. Most of them were raised in either working- or middle-class families, while a small number were raised in conditions of extreme poverty. As expected, only one Latino gay man came from an opulent family. The category of change, one row before the last, refers to those who went through changes in class position while growing up. Among those in Chicago, two changed from middle class to poor and working class respectively. Another activist described a move that went from working class to middle class and then to a situation in which the family struggled financially. Among activists in San Francisco, three described upward mobility. One moved from poor to middle class and two from working to middle class. The fourth activist described a decline in social class, from working class to poor.

Table 1. Distribution of Social Class Position from Growing Up to Adulthood by City Among Latino GBT Activists*

Social class	Growing Up			Adulthood		
	Chicago	San Francisco	Total	Chicago	San Francisco	Total
Poor	5	5	10	9	15	24
Working class	19	16	35	16	9	25
Middle class	12	13	25	15	14	29
Wealthy	0	1	1	0	1	1
Change	3	4	7	0	0	0
Total	39	39	78	40	39	79

*Totals do not add up to 80 because of missing information.

The data on current social-class position indicate that, as a group, these GBTs experienced a downward mobility since growing up. Notably, some who grew up in working-class families are currently living in poverty. This pattern is clearer among those living in San Francisco than among those in Chicago. The data do not account for the causes of downward mobility, but two factors seem to be related to poverty in the adult years. One is living with HIV. Eight HIV-positive activists in San Francisco and six in Chicago live in poverty. Most of them are not employed and live on public assistance. The second factor related to adult poverty is lacking legal residence in the United States. In San Francisco, for instance, four volunteers and activists living in poverty do not have legal documents, which could help them in seeking jobs and social services.

It must be noted that there is still some variation within each of those four categories. In the middle class, for instance, it is possible to further group activists into upper and lower-middle factions. For efficiency and clarity, however, I keep the five-category classification. Next, I present examples from the four main categories. I selected examples based on richness (e.g., breadth and detail of the narrative) and representativeness. I also aimed for diversity in terms of country or region of origin (e.g., United States, Central America, South America). The Latino GBTs interviewed and the vignettes presented are not representative samples—hence, generalizations may not be appropriate. Yet, the sample comprises adequate variability in terms of social class-class. The vignettes illustrate the range of experiences narrated by these activists.

The Poor

The stories of *compañeros* who grew up in poverty frequently refer to an arduous childhood, plagued by worries about not having food and clothing. As children, many of them worked in the fields and farms. Toys and other diversions are absent from their stories. Their narratives evoke dark and melancholy scenes of small enclosed spaces and vast distances. These GBTs grew up in overcrowded rooms that didn't allow them to enjoy the notion of a bedroom or a living room. They lived in the outskirts of cities or in public housing projects, away from basic services such as drinkable water, public transportation, and schools. They also had to move continually— from one house to another, from a town to a city, and from one country to another—in search of a living. Ultimately, these activists saw themselves as different from the better-off children. The better-off children had all they lacked: a house, cars, and light skin color.

Jimmy

Jimmy describes his first years as "a very difficult childhood." He was raised by a single mother in a rural area of central Mexico in the early 1970s. His mother had six children. Three of his siblings migrated to Mexico City in search of jobs when Jimmy was born. His mother then had a boy and a girl after Jimmy.

> I never got presents for Christmas or Santos Reyes [Epiphany]. Also, I never had enough school supplies, like pens and colored pencils. I had to work when I was little—when I was four years old. I used to watch the turkeys, keeping them in the pen. I'd get some money and then my mother would buy me a box of colored pencils for the year. I lacked many things. I saw my mother getting desperate, because sometimes there was nothing to eat. Sometimes I'd go to school hungry. We'd eat only once a day. At age of 15 I began working full-time.

Jimmy's father lived in the same town. He had an affair with Jimmy's mother while married to another woman, with whom he already had children. He never provided for Jimmy. Two of Jimmy's half-siblings went to the same school as Jimmy. "His sons had nice school supplies, like colored notebooks. I'd stare at them. I wanted a notebook like theirs, but it was expensive." Jimmy's mother worked in the fields. She used to arrange for landlords and managers to hire Jimmy on a weekly or monthly basis to watch the animals:

> I'd do both, school and work. And when the teachers asked for supplies for school projects, what was I supposed to do? I had no alternative but to get up at dawn, go to work, and then to school by 8 o'clock. Then go to work again after school. I'd do my homework in the bus, hungry. My mother worried a lot.

Jimmy did not attend high school. Later in his life, he and two brothers emigrated to the United States. First he lived in New York City, where he became HIV positive. He now lives in Chicago. At the time of our conversation, Jimmy was looking for a job and taking vocational training courses.

Gabriel

"I really didn't have a childhood," Gabriel recounts about his early years spent with his mother in the strawberry fields of California. He was born in Mexico, but his family emigrated to California shortly after his birth in 1973. His father first worked in a factory for a couple years. When the factory closed, he went back to do farm work. Gabriel was subsequently raised by two farmworkers—or, as he says, "campesinos":

> I was born in Mexico. I lived there for like maybe six months to a year. My family emigrated to this country in 1973. I was an infant. So I have no recollection

of Mexico. I was raised in North Salinas. . . . In the early '70s, there were very few Latinos, so in Salinas we were one of the first big Latino families in my area. I remember bilingual education was getting introduced and I remember how I used to get pulled out of my classes because I didn't speak English.

I went to an almost-all-white elementary school, because there were not a lot of Latinos. No Blacks, no Asians, just white. We used to live in this low-income, huge, four-bedroom apartment in Salinas, but now I see the apartment at this age and it looks really small.

So then my dad lost his job. My father used to work for this really lucrative company, but it broke down. We had to move to East Salinas. Of course, it's very different from North Salinas. It was like East LA or East San Jose. It was all Mexicans. No Central Americans. No South Americans. Just Mexicans. I didn't meet other Latinos until I went to college. I didn't even know how they looked. Then [in East Salinas], I went to a different elementary school, full of Mexican kids. I wasn't used to it. It was like a little culture shock.

Gabriel was eight years old when his father lost his job, changing the family's financial situation slightly. Before, the family was, in Gabriel's words, "low income" and continued to live as such once the father returned to farmwork. This resulted in changes in Gabriel's neighborhood, schooling, and peers. He notes the stark contrast between the neighborhoods in particular:

So I think it had more of an impact in terms of just the living . . . of going to an all-Mexican school. . . . I was scared. *Cholos* and gangsters. When we lived in North Salinas, we used to always watch the news. "Otra muerte" [Another death]. "Balacearon a fulano" [They shot a guy]. "They stabbed a guy."

It was a lot dirtier on the East Side. Things weren't well kept. People had fences. On the North Side people didn't have fences. People had more trust. It was more open. People mowed their lawns, people weeded their gardens. People had gardens, flowers. People walked their dogs. Nice dogs like poodles or fucking Chihuahuas. On the East Side, people walked their dogs, but they weren't poodles or Chihuahuas. They were pit bulls, Dobermans . . . mean dogs, mutts.

East Salinas had a lot of convenient stores within the community and *taquerias.* Where in North Salinas, if you wanted to go to a convenient store, you would go to Quick-Stop or 7-Eleven.

Images of strawberry fields permeate Gabriel's childhood memories. When he was five, his mother took him and his four siblings to work with her in the fields. This left a sour memory, as he disliked the physical labor, could not play as other boys did, and endured the taunts of other children. Yet this harsh experience and his brother's encouragement inspired Gabriel to leave Salinas and go to college and "be somebody":

I just remember . . . working in the strawberry fields. My mom started taking me around five, but I wasn't really picking yet. Since I was really small, I would be in the same *surco* [furrow] with my mom. I was in front of her or in back of her. Of course, she's picking really fast, and I'll just pick one or two and just kind of help her.

But once I was old enough, my mom had me working and I stopped working when I was 14. I hated it so much because I didn't really have a childhood. Kids that don't work after school, they watch TV, they play with their friends, on weekends they sleep in, they watch cartoons, they go swimming, they go to basketball camps. Well, not me . . . Saturday morning, 7:00, fields. It was dark out. It was cold, foggy . . . The *brisa* [breeze] . . . and you had to go pick to supplement the family income.

"OK, how can I escape this?" By staying in school and being a good student. I want to be somebody. My dad is a *campesino*. "I don't want to be a *campesino*, I can do much more."

Plus, we were all really good in school, all six of us. So, all of us worked in the fields. [I hated] that our hands used to turn black and blue and red . . . and your hands would be stained. Then you would go to school and kids would make fun of you. I would always hide my hands like this [making a fist].

Gabriel worked in the fields through his teenage years. He could not live or do as better-off teenagers could. Then, his older brother earned a scholarship and went to college in the northeast, defying his parents' wishes. This opened up Gabriel's prospects to get a college degree, explore the outside world, and move out of poverty:

As a teenager, my older brother was in college . . . He was important to me because he would write to me, and I would write back. He went to school on the East Coast. He ran away from home, basically, to go to school. My father was angered, not very thrilled, and upset. My mom knew he was going to go. My mom was like, "No te vayas, tu papá se va enojar" [Don't go, your dad is going to get upset]. "Me voy, mama, me voy" [I'm leaving, Mom, I'm leaving].

During that time I was an eighth grader and he was a freshman in college, he would write to me. He would say, "Oh my God, I'm going to need so much. I want you to do the same. God, it's just so much more than Salinas." I didn't know what he was talking about, all I knew was Salinas. It was like living in a cage. That's why I left Salinas.

Gabriel chose to move to San Francisco. After finishing college he went back to Salinas and at age twenty-five, moved to the Bay Area, where he enjoys a more comfortable life than when he was a child. He has a full-time job with the state government, has a car, and provides some financial support to his parents.

George

George is a thirty-seven-year-old gay man living in Chicago. He grew up on the outskirts of one of the largest metropolitan areas of Mexico. His father worked in an upholstery shop but suffered from alcoholism. He spent most of his income on alcohol. His mother worked in the informal economy, selling clothes and crafts. She sold clothes that her brother sent to her from the United States. George's parents, brother, and sister lived with his mother's parents until George was a teenager. For George, it is not easy to talk about his childhood, as he says, "It is unpleasant. . . . It's unpleasant to remember all of that." He faced material deprivation, his father's alcoholism and abuse of his mother, and discrimination from his middle-class school peers:

> We lived with my mom's parents. We were poor. We all lived in one little room. The house had two bedrooms, a dining room, the kitchen, and in the back it had an apartment, where my mom's brother lived with his family. My grandparents slept in one bedroom and we all in the other room. Back then there were my mom, dad, my brother, and my little sister.
>
> The barrio was poor, outside the city. All the *colonias* [neighborhoods] in the area were poor. There was no pavement. There was no drinking water. We had to walk about two blocks to get water and shower. We had to bring water in buckets. The buses would come, but about every hour only. To go to the city you needed the whole day.
>
> I went to an elementary school that was about 10 blocks from home. When I finished, my dad sent me to a school far away. Supposedly, because it was a very good school. Despite the fact that I was the effeminate and mannered of the family, my dad always saw me as the smart one. He said, "because you're smart, I'll send you to a good school."
>
> The school was in the other side of the city. It was an expedition every day to go to junior high school. I'd take three different buses. It was a one-hour trip. That school was sort of traumatic for me because the kids there were upper middle class, and I was poor. I'd see them with their nice shining shoes and good clothes. They were *güeritos* [little whites] and I was *más moreno* [darker] than them. In Mexico, there is social-class discrimination. There is also discrimination when they see you [are] *más moreno* [darker] or *más bajito* [shorter].

When George was in junior high school, his parents bought a small lot and began building some rooms. They moved out of his grandparents'. A few years later, when George was nineteen years old, his father left the family. George did not finish high school. Instead, he moved to Chicago, where his uncle lived, and looked to improve his financial situation and support his mother. George sent money to his mother, enabling her to finish the house ten years after they had moved in.

The Working Class

The accounts of those *compañeros* from working-class families offer some subtle variations on the themes encountered among those who grew up in poverty. While some of them mention the persistent economic hardships that they have faced, others make no mention of such difficulties and even talk about a happy childhood. The images in these stories are not entirely gray or clouded. They contain hints of brightness and color. Nature is not always an adversary. At times it is a playmate. In these stories, basic needs are met and there is time and space for play. School is accessible and a source of a few warm memories, particularly when the discussion turns to the feeling of pride that comes with getting good grades. Children enjoy extracurricular activities, such as dance and sports. Instead of cardboard houses, there are houses made of brick, which provide a firm footing. Yet, limiting and crowded living spaces are still present, along with public housing and divisive and dangerously close train tracks.

Mario

"It was not a well-off home, but a home in which we never lacked anything." This is how Mario assesses the financial situation of his family when he was growing up in Central America. He is the fifth of eight children. Five of these children, including Mario, come from the first marriage of Mario's father. Mario's parents divorced when he was about one year old, but the father kept the children and then remarried. Mario regards his father's second wife as his mother. His father had a marble shop, and his mother was a schoolteacher:

> My dad was something of an artist. He supported the family working in the marble business. We didn't have everything, because we were many. . . . But my parents let me do everything. I did classical dance when I was 11. I also was in a national folk dance group. In elementary school, I was in a play, as Peter Pan. My mother, that is, my father's wife, was a schoolteacher. She also made some money sewing, like dresses and wedding dresses.

Mario went to college, completed his degree, and then got married. From that marriage he now has two teenagers. Later, he divorced and came to San Francisco, where he works as a nurse. Mario just celebrated his fiftieth birthday. As implied above, he thinks highly of his parents and is thankful for how they raised him. He has fond memories of his childhood and has tried to pass on to his children the values and worldview he learned from his parents:

Everybody in the block had a business or was selling something. The woman next door had a store. The guy across the street had a mill. He ground corn. The woman on the other side of the house sold firewood. Then, another guy made ice cream. Next door to him was the barbershop and after that a small diner, where an old lady cooked and sold food. By the corner, there was the woman who made tortillas. Next it was the shoe shop and then an old man who packed candy to sell in the stores. And my father was the marble guy.

There was also a river, close by. The river was dirty, but in the river there were these trees that had a sweet fruit. We'd jump, climb up the trees, and eat lots of fruits.

But something very important I grew up with is that we, the children, weren't expected to help our parents out. Nothing like, "I send money to my mom" or "my father needs my money to eat." It might sound rude, but my father used to say, "You worry about your own families." I'm the same way. I don't expect my children to take care of me. I raised them so that they could fly and stumble.

Armando

Armando works in the social-services industry in the Bay Area. He is twenty-five years old, went to college on the East Coast with a full scholarship, and currently attends part-time graduate school. He comes, however, from a financially modest family with three children. As he notes, "I always kind of identified with the working class. We never lacked the basic necessities." His father is a mechanic and has worked in factories most of his life. Originally from Mexico, he did not finish elementary school. He has had a drinking problem as long as Armando can remember. Armando's mother has worked part-time, intermittently. The salient circumstance in his childhood narrative is the repeated moves back and forth between central Mexico and Southern California:

> I was actually born and raised in both Mexico and Santa Ana, which is near Los Angeles. When I was little, my parents moved around a lot. I went to five different elementary schools, including two years in Mexico. My mom had me when she was 17. She got married at 15. But they were great parents. . . . At the same time, they were pretty traumatic in some instances. Like my dad's still an alcoholic, and he beat my mom a lot.
>
> I remember sweet things in Mexico, like hanging out with my great-grandma in the farms. We'd go to pick oranges up. We had lots of parties and I met many cousins. It was just beautiful. I remember having a lot of fun.

When Armando was ten years old, his parents left him in Los Angeles with his father's parents. Once more, his parents went to Mexico. With space tight at his grandparents' home because three of Armando's aunts also lived there along with an uncle and his family, Armando slept on the floor in his aunts' bedroom. Yet Armando preferred to stay in the United States, "I remember at ten not wanting to go back to Mexico with my mom because I knew I didn't have a future down there." Armando explains that he was always good at school and that his grades, as well as the support of his aunt, helped him get to college. He was among the top students in his high school. His Aunt Luisa, who was in the same high school and a couple of years older than Armando, was the first of her family to attend college. She encouraged Armando to follow in her footsteps. While in high school he became a frequent user of marijuana and acid, but he stopped using them when he went to college:

> I've always been good at school, and I've always gotten so much support from teachers. Ultimately, that's one of the things that saved me. Sometimes I think, "God, if I didn't have straight A's and didn't have the grades to go to college . . . what would have become of me? I wouldn't be me."
>
> I just wanted to learn things. I wanted to be successful in life. I wanted to have material things at that time. Like I saw my friends driving really nice cars that their parents bought for them. And I said, "Wow! Will I ever have that?"
>
> I think most of it just came from my inner self. I won a lot of speech awards in high school. I got awards for math, because I was always good in math. I think I got first place in math one year. I have so many trophies, even tennis trophies. I was number one singles in my whole high school in my senior year. I was ranked among the top ten in the whole state. Part of me thinks if I'd have had a coach and the money, I think I would have had a chance to become very good.

Ivan

Despite being raised by a single mother and in public housing, Ivan has pleasant memories of his childhood. "My childhood was colorful," he notes in reference to his days in one of the largest public housing neighborhoods in Puerto Rico. His mother worked as a secretary to support Ivan and his two sisters. His parents divorced when Ivan was two years old. Ivan's father was a government employee and provided child support, but it was insufficient for the three children:

> I was raised in a barrio, in a public housing area, where there were all sorts of people from different walks of life. I always went to public schools and had very good grades. I was dedicated and kind of quiet. But I also loved the street. I broke a leg once, then an arm.
>
> Although it was public housing, the community was united. Everybody knew each other. Like in the morning, you'd hear, "Mrs. Juana, you got any sugar? I have the coffee ready." We never locked the doors. The women neighbors were always looking after us. It was a nice childhood.

Ivan is thirty-five years old and now lives in Chicago. He started college but has not yet finished. He is working in the health care industry. His mother has retired and still lives in Puerto Rico. Ivan's sisters do as well as he does.

Ernesto

"My childhood was a bit difficult, let's say, it is the childhood of many kids back in my country during the war." These are the words thirty-five-year-old Ernesto uses as he begins telling the story of his life. He was born in a Central American country, just before a civil war erupted. The war had a collective impact on Ernesto and his family:

> I grew up in the war. This marks you somewhat, because as a kid you see all these soldiers and you begin to fear them. But then, it was a normal situation for me. I remember in the mornings, when my father would bring the newspaper, reading, "In such place, 15 killed." "In this other place, 5 killed in a clash." "The priest of this place killed by paramilitaries."

Ernesto comes from a working-class family. Both of his parents worked, but his mother worked from home, as she raised thirteen children. During the war, however, the family struggled financially as they were forced to move, losing their home and income. Ernesto's father was an evangelical minister for a church that helped the family through this time:

> When I was three years old, we moved to the other side of the country because of the war. We arrived at the doorsteps of my father's church in the capital. We had a suitcase with clothes and some kitchen utensils. That was all.
>
> We got there and a church brother told us about the lots the church had outside the city. We got there and built a room with cardboard. It was a shack. We lived there for a year. We moved because it rained a lot and the harvest wasn't good. I will never forget it. I remember very well when my mother had my little sister. The house would get all wet. Because it'd never stop raining. My father hung a plastic sheet on top of my mother's bed, so that she and my little sister wouldn't get wet. Then my father would empty the plastic sheet, bailing the water out with a large bowl.
>
> Then we moved closer to the city. We built a house with bamboo sticks and sheet metal. My father got a job in the government. We were able to put down a brick floor.

Several months later, Ernesto's parents set up a small store in front of their house. Ernesto's mother took care of the store while his father worked, usually through midnight. They saved some money, bought a lot in a better neighborhood, and began building a house:

Then, we set up a small store, like a pantry. The problem with that house was that it was right by the train tracks. My dad always worried we would [get] run over by a train. So with the store and my dad's job, they saved some money to buy a lot in a safer area. At home, we have always worked. He used to say that home was like enterprise, we all have to invest in it to gain.

Ernesto is HIV positive. He did not finish high school and has not met his two younger siblings, who were born after he moved to Chicago. He has only seen pictures of them. Ernesto's living situation is very precarious. He lives in a supported-living unit and makes extra money cleaning tables during the weekends.

The Middle Class

Having a middle-class status means, primarily, access to resources and freedom of movement. The parents in these stories are business owners and professionals. They have not one but two or three houses, and they are interested in their children's education. The images conveyed in the stories are of wide-open, colorful spaces. Living quarters are not crowded. Children and teenagers have their own rooms. They can move freely between social classes. They can also travel, not for living, but for vacation to the beach and overseas. Absent from these accounts is concern about meeting basic needs. Instead, we find an interest in well-being, safety, reducing stress, and attending college.

Fabian

Fabian grew up in a large Mexican industrial city. Born in 1964, he has a brother and a sister, and his parents owned a business. Both of his parents were members of one of the socialist parties in the country; hence, Fabian's upbringing was shaped by his parents' political activism and ideas about social class and social change, as is evident in his narrative:

> My parents always were interested in our getting a good education. But I think we felt differently because we were atheist and my father was a Communist. Many people don't understand what communism is. He had very progressive ideas, but back then you couldn't speak loudly because of political repression.
>
> My parents come from humble families. They come from small towns. They had to work very hard. They are self-taught people. They love to read, and they are very smart. But they also had aspirations of moving up . . . That's good, but it can also hurt you because it's like self-rejection -not accepting yourself.
>
> But both of my parents are very kind. They are idealists. They believe in a better world, in the ideal that there will no be social-class contradictions, that

poverty will end, that all will be better. My dad used to say, "You'll see the day Mexico becomes a socialist country. The day when there will be education for everybody and there will be no poor people."

Fabian attended public schools from kindergarten through college, where he earned a degree in civil engineering. He also went to music school and traveled throughout Mexico as a child. Fabian recalls two close child-hood friends, one who was middle-class, like him, and the other who was working-class:

> My friend Aldo was very ingenious. We'd chat about music, because we were in music school together. We'd pretend to have a radio program. Then, my friend Rico was the other side of me, my wild side. Rico was a kid from a low social class. He was terrible. He was adventurous. I was the good boy. Rico was the bad kid. He had bad grades and was naughty. But we were always together.
>
> When I was little, we lived in a poor neighborhood. At age six or seven, we moved to a middle-class neighborhood, where middle-class people wanted to pass as upper-class. So, when I wasn't with Aldo, who lived in the same middle-class neighborhood, I was with my friends in the poor neighborhood only four blocks away. These friends were untamed. . . . It was an escape for me from the pressure of being a model kid.

In his late twenties, Fabian married and moved with his wife to Chicago, where he worked for a construction firm. After a couple of years, the mar-riage failed. Now, Fabian lives with his boyfriend in a small house they bought together.

Ismael

"In Mexico," Ismael explains, "your social status is measured by how many maids you have. It might sound insulting, but it's about how many cleaning ladies you can afford and what school your children attend." In Mexico, Ismael's family had a staff of five people in the house and owned several houses, including a vacation home. His father ran a business and his mother managed the properties. Ismael's social-class background is more accurately characterized as upper-middle-class because, as he elaborates, his parents were not wealthy and both of them worked:

> I was born in a home with my father, my mother, and three siblings. My home was financially stable. We had people to help in the house, several cars, and a nice house with several bedrooms. I went to the best private school in the city, a Catholic school.
>
> But then my father decided to come to the States with his brother. Following my father, we came to Chicago a year after my father got here.

When the family arrived in Chicago, the mother joined the father work-ing in a small factory. Yet, they kept some of their Mexican properties, which they rented out. Soon Ismael's parents were able to set up their own business and buy a house in Chicago. During this time, Ismael continued his education in a private Catholic school. The family lived in Chicago for several years and then returned to Mexico, except for the father. The stay in Mexico, however, was short, as Ismael's mother decided to come back to the United States a year later. This time, it was permanent.

Ismael's mother did not work in Mexico. The family lived off the proper-ties they kept and the father's income. When Ismael finished junior high, he was sent to a public school. Then, he obtained an associate's degree and currently works full-time for a health insurance company while attending college. He plans to attend medical school. He and his boyfriend of three years recently bought a condominium.

Bernardo

Bernardo is a thirty-nine-year-old engineer living outside of San Francisco. He owns the townhouse he lives in as well as a small cabin in Northern California. Bernardo grew up in a northern Mexican border city. Both of his parents worked, his father in the tourism industry and his mother cleaned homes across the border. They earned their income in dollars, which allowed them a relatively comfortable life in Mexico. "I liked my childhood," Bernardo says of his early years. Bernardo and his brother at-tended public schools in Mexico but went to college in the United States, as was the custom among many Mexican middle-class and well-off students along the northern border:

> We had a house. My dad had bought the land and built a house when I was about two. I'd say it was a middle-class neighborhood. It was a three-bedroom house with enough land. We had pets, like peacocks and dogs, and lots of plants. It was a good and safe neighborhood . . .

As Bernardo continues, he expands on what he sees as two significant events in his life. The first is when his father bought him his first car. The second even is when he went to college. His father wanted him to study medicine, but Bernardo was not interested:

> I got my first car when I was 18. My dad bought it for me and that was kind of nice. It was my last year in high school. I wanted a big Granada. My dad and I were shopping for cars for a while and then there was one that I saw that I really liked. My dad was negotiating. He was a man that would never buy anything through credit, and it was like $3,200 or $3,300.

Every day, I would take the bus from the high school to home. I would pass by the car lot and see it to make sure that it was still there. Then, one day, it wasn't, and I went home and my dad said, "We should go and check out the car again," and I said, "You know what? It's gone." He goes, "Yes, that's too bad . . ." And I said, "Yes, because I really liked that one." Then he gave me the key and said, "It was in the back. They're cleaning it up for you." It was the first car I ever had. I had it for about five years and took it to college.

In my second year in high school I got focused more on college. I remember a friend of my brother recommended this book called *Career Guide,* something like that. It was a really cool book. It had every single career you could do in Mexico. So it had all kinds of engineering, medicine, and so on. I wanted to study history, but I knew my dad wouldn't go for it, and he was paying for college. I liked engineering also, and I knew it was a career that I could make a career out of it after college, so I did that.

I thought I will study anything as long as I can get away from town or get away from the house. Luckily, the local college didn't have civil engineering, I knew I had to go out of town. That's what I wanted. I wanted to go to Mexico City because I felt I wanted to go to a big city. My grandmother didn't like the idea. She said, "It's too far away, there's so much crime there." She hadn't been there in decades. One of my cousins had gone to the States, and I followed that precedent.

Angelica

Angelica spent her childhood in three countries, United States, Italy, and Mexico, because her father worked in foreign service. Her father is of European descent and her mother is of Mexican descent. Angelica was born in the United States, but when she was three, the family moved to Mexico. After several years there, the family moved to Rome, where they lived three years. Then, the family returned to the United States. Because of the father's job, the family enjoyed many amenities, more than they could otherwise have afforded, especially while living abroad. The family was provided with house staff and a chauffeur, and the children had access to the best private schools. In her story, Angelica contrasts two worlds, abroad in the foreign service and United States suburbia:

> Those memories are really beautiful. My dad worked for the foreign service. Even though we didn't make a lot of money, I went to private schools with like oil kids, internationals, and movie stars' kids. . . . Then after he retired, we went to middle-class America. I thought it was really cool, 'cause I never had a sink that had just one faucet where you could control the hot and cold water. So to me it was like, wow! And carpet everywhere.
>
> I was too young to really notice, but culturally it was a really great experience. I learned languages. I spoke Italian when I was there. I still understand

it, read it, and speak it. . . . But also 'cause I grew up in a big city, you don't just walk outside and hang out with your friends. All has to be arranged. Like, they call their mom and someone picks them up, or you get driven over to their apartment.

Then when we moved back to the States. It was my first suburban experience. I was actually really happy, because I got to live in Alexandria [Virginia]. And the houses are really nice. Like they're all colonial style. I had neighbor kids to play with. I really liked it. . . . Well, actually, I didn't like my school, 'cause they would tease me a lot 'cause I didn't speak English like everyone else did. And I was really feminine and I dressed funny, too. 'Cause I dressed European.

The year after their return, the family moved to a suburb in Northern California. There, Angelica finished high school, in a public school. She did not go to college right after that. As she puts it, "I didn't care. I didn't think about getting into college." By that time, Angelica was using cocaine and acid, and experimenting with cross-dressing. She then moved to San Francisco, where now she attends design school and makes her living designing clothes.

The Wealthy

Simon is the only *compañero* who grew up in an opulent environment. A sixty-four-year-old gay man originally from Central America, he has lived in San Francisco for nearly twenty years. Both of his parents come from well-to-do immigrant families. His grandparents came from Western Europe and owned several haciendas in Central America. Simon's childhood took place against a backdrop of a large home, a nanny, and chauffeurs. When he finished elementary school, Simon was sent to an elite preparatory school in the United States in accordance with the family's expectations. His father and mother also had attended college in the United States. Simon's life, however, was altered by a civil war in his country:

> I was born in a house with 11 maids. My parents and my grandparents were millionaires. My house was huge and had a very large patio. I remember play-ing baseball inside the house and roller-skating in the hallways. We lived with my grandpa and my two sisters.
>
> Since I was very little, I knew I was going to be sent to a military academy in the United States. Since I was a little boy I was arrogant. I knew I was pretty and smart, and I knew I had lots of money and status. I had my own nanny. I went to private schools and I was always neatly dressed all in white. A chauf-feur drove me to school all the time.
>
> So I finished elementary school and then came here to the United States. I went from the military academy to college and, then, I did some studies in France. I returned to New York and started living between the two countries—my

home country where my mother lived, and here. Then war came. We lost a lot of stuff. I left to Mexico, where I lived for two years. I returned home, but it was difficult to live with my mother. . . . I moved to San Francisco.

Life amid such wealth did not make Simon happy. Reflecting on his life, he says that he is now more content than before, despite living with HIV and in a modest middle-class position:

> My happiness has always been strange. It is an ambiguous term. Having it all, I wasn't happy. I lived better than 99 percent of the people in Latin America and I was never happy. I was never happy in Latin America. That's why I'm here.

Most of these volunteers and activists grew up in working- and middle-class milieus. A small group of them grew up in poverty, and only one of them came from a wealthy family. Those who lived in poverty as children usually gave accounts of a difficult childhood or of not having a childhood at all. The stories of their lives are about overcoming the adversities that arise from class and race sociopolitical systems. In contrast, those who come from working- or middle-class backgrounds often spoke about being happy as children and having the basic necessities for life. The social class in which these men were raised shaped their lives as adults. It influenced their access to assets, such as education and skills. It also shaped their access to health, play, and travel. Some of the men who grew up in working-class families experienced declining mobility as adults. A significant number of them are currently living in poverty. Two factors seem to affect such a trajectory. One is the deterioration of their health due to HIV and AIDS. The other is their immigration to the United States with no legal status. In the following chapters, we will see in detail how their lives have unfolded.

CHAPTER TWO

GENDER DEVIANTS

"Cucurrucucu, paloma. Cucurrucucu, no llores" (dove, don't cry), Blanca sang to me as she described the night a promoter found her singing in a nightclub. "Cucurrucucu Paloma," a ranchera song, was made popular by Lola Beltrán, known in Mexico as the "queen of ranchero music." In the early 1960s, at the age of twenty-five, Blanca took the stage persona of Lola Beltrán and started making her living singing in bars and nightclubs in California. She frequently used the word *queen* to describe herself, instead of the longer *drag queen*. She was very proud of her gifted voice, which, according to her, many compared to Beltrán's. She could not make it as a singer, however, because she was not a "real" woman.

> Back then, you had to be honest to Mexican audiences. If you were passing as a woman and then revealed you were a man, it was a fraud. The only place I could sing and be Lola Beltrán was in a nightclub for effeminate men.

Ironically, Blanca's talent was also her affliction, as she crossed the gender boundaries set up by her society and her times. "Yo sufrí mucho" (I suffered a lot), she says of her early years in Southern California. Both of her Mexican parents were very religious. Her mother was Catholic and her father Pentecostal. Blanca was frequently scolded for what her parents and older brothers perceived as womanlike behavior. As a child, she used to play putting on her aunt's dresses and lipstick. The kids in the neighborhood made fun of her, but she did not care. She enjoyed wearing the dresses. Her aunt did not mind and even defended her. She would tell Blanca's mother not to beat her. "He is *joto* [faggot], and that's the way he is. God sent him to you—accept him." While on one of the weekend visits to her aunt, Blanca had sex with a seventeen-year-old cousin. "I was a child but didn't say anything. I let him do it." Blanca, speaking in a-matter-of-fact manner, explains that she did not try to stop the cousin because a part of her longed for sexual contact with a man. Blanca did not finish elementary school because she was "traumatized." Children in the school would pick on her and sexually harass her, to the point that it became intolerable and Blanca stopped going to school. When she was eleven years old, Blanca was sent to a psychiatric hospital. One of her older brothers persuaded the parents that she was mentally ill and needed to be cured and made into a "normal man." Initially, she was in the hospital for three months. The doctors told the parents she was not mentally ill and that there was nothing to be cured. Blanca's father, however, refused to take her back, and she ended up staying four years. Soon after she left the hospital, Blanca left her family. Years later, she settled in San Francisco, where she became a community figure thanks to her talent as a "queen" singer. A year after I interviewed her, Blanca died from AIDS-related complications. She was living in a transitional home for homeless people.

Blanca's life was marked by the stigma attached to gender nonconforming behavior. As defined by Goffman (1963), stigma is the labeling of individuals or groups in a way that discredits them. Stigma is a social process by which a dominant group negatively labels a condition (e.g., homosexual desire) that deviates from the group's standards of normality. This labeling involves the assignation of undesirable characteristics (e.g., weak, perverse, dirty), a social separation or distancing, and the use of discriminatory practices toward those labeled as "different" (Link and Phelan 2001; Link et al. 1997; Meyer 1995; Ramirez-Valles et al. 2005). Gay and transgender people, thus, are stigmatized because they deviate from the dominant gender ideology and threaten that same gender ideology or social order. In Blanca's case, she was labeled as different because her thoughts, desires, and actions did not correspond to what her family, neighbors, and larger society expected from someone with a penis. She was labeled a "joto," thought to be mentally ill, institutionalized, beaten and reprimanded, and used as a sexual object.

Stigmatized persons may experience stigma in the form of acts such as name-calling, social rejection, or job discrimination. They may be aware that society (e.g., family members, employers, religious groups) harbors negative beliefs and attitudes toward them; therefore, they may feel forced to act in ways as to avoid negative consequences. Perhaps the most damaging aspect of stigma is its internalization—that is, when stigmatized persons incorporate the negative attributes created by the dominant group into their own self-concept (Fife and Wright 2000; Link et al. 1997; Ramirez-Valles et al. 2005).

The stigma toward gender nonconformity may have profound negative consequences for many LGBT persons. Such stigma may lead to suicide, unemployment, and low self-esteem (Cochran and Mays 2000; Link and

Phelan 2001; Mays and Cochran 2001; Paul et al. 2002; Frable et al. 1997; Huebner et al. 2002; Williamson 2000; Meyer 1995; Turner et al. 1993). Unfortunately, the AIDS epidemic intensified this stigma (Herek 1999). From the start of the epidemic in the 1980s, the scientific and popular discourse equated HIV/AIDS with homosexual behavior among men.

Although stigma has decreased in the United States and Latin America (Loftus 2001; Carrillo 2002), the majority of LGBT people continue experiencing it (Díaz and Ayala 2001; Kaiser Family Foundation 2001). Gay and transgender people are no longer institutionalized, as Blanca was in 1950s; however, many of them are still sent to psychologists and psychiatrists, called names, assaulted, harassed, and socially rejected, as I show in this chapter.

In this chapter I examine *compañeros'* experiences of stigmatization related to their nonconforming gender behavior. Their life stories allow us to see, with the benefit of retrospection, how stigma works. As in Blanca's story, they provide insight not only into the type of stigmatizing experiences (e.g., name-calling, social rejection), but also into the sources, consequences, and strategies used to cope with—and confront—stigma. Collectively, the life stories show that childhood is the period in which most stigmatization is experienced—and perhaps causes the most lasting consequences. At this time in life, family and school are the most salient sources of stigma, as they are the main socializing agents. Some of these *compañeros* internalized such stigma, but most of them have been able to overcome the internalization in the course of their lives. Yet, they speak of depression, failed suicide attempts, and dislocation as consequences of the stigma they endured. The experienced stigma and its consequences are particularly severe for those activists who identify as drag queens (like Blanca), transexual, or transgender. Since they were children, their actions were perceived by others as flagrant transgressions of gender norms.

In the Family

One of the first life domains children are socialized into is gender roles. The family constitutes the primary learning source. From an early age, children learn that behaviors, such as tone of voice and the way of walking, games, and clothes are categorized as being either for boys or girls. There is no surprise, then, to find that most of the stigma experienced by GBTs originates in the family during their childhood. "We all get discriminated against," Salvador says. "I'm not the only one." As children, these men learned that actions and thoughts that do not conform to their assigned gender are labeled abnormal and are punished. The punishment comes in different forms, ranging from name-calling to beating. Mainly, parents carry out punishment. But siblings, aunts, and grandparents are also prone to stigmatizing.

Recounting his early years, Salvador says, "My family has always rejected me, because of who I am. . . . At age of five, I didn't consider myself a normal boy." When Salvador was about six years old, he was having sex with his older brothers and was playing with dolls. As a result, he was frequently called "maricón" (sissy), beaten by his father, and rejected by most family members. In Mexico, where Salvador was raised in the mid-1970s, *maricón* is a pejorative used to label a man whose behavior is perceived as woman-like. Salvador had eleven siblings, including four older brothers with whom he regularly shared beds. He first started having oral sex with the eldest brother. "I longed to touch his penis." Salvador's sexual relations with his brothers went on for a couple of years, until his father became aware of them. His father then demanded that Salvador's mother "put this boy apart because he's doing his *chingaderas* [dirty things] with his brothers."

Salvador's sexual relations, however, were not the only behavior that his family deemed disturbing. He liked to put on his mother's dresses. One day, an older brother caught him. Upset, the brother yelled, "If I ever find out that you're *maricón*, I'll kill you." "I'll never forget it," Salvador says, alluding to the pain and rejection that he still feels.

Salvador also liked playing with dolls. In an attempt to change Salvador's behavior, the father would buy him marbles, which boys customarily play with in Mexico. Salvador would throw the marbles away and secretively continue to play with his sisters' dolls. When his father found out, he reprimanded and beat Salvador. In another painfully remembered incident, Salvador was beaten by his father for not challenging the kids who ridiculed him. Salvador and his parents were walking through the neighborhood when a couple of boys called him *maricón* and made fun of the way he was walking. "Look how he wiggles his hips," they taunted. The father heard the comments and told Salvador that he would beat him up if Salvador did not strike those kids. "Now you have to act like a man," his father ordered. "He beat me so hard that I haven't forgotten it," Salvador recalled. Even his sisters picked on Salvador's walking. They called him *señorita* (miss) and did not want to hang out with him for fear of being stigmatized:

> My sisters said, "Look, Mom, how he walks." They'd tell me, "When you're with us, you have to walk straight, like a man." I'd feel bad. I'd try to act macho. My sisters would tell me: "What would our dates think if we have a *joto* brother?"

Salvador's experiences point to the existence of a particularly dominant gender social system which is reproduced by and in the family, as it exercises control over its members. The name-calling, scolding, physical mistreatment, and rejection experienced by Salvador were the result of his nonconforming gender actions, which are referred to by many *compañeros* as "mannerisms," "the way I was," "not normal," and "obvious." They were also problematic because they threatened the family's image. The reactions of his father, brothers, and sisters are based on a fear of being labeled as "the family with *joto* son" or "the brother/sister of the *joto*." There is a preoccupation among family members to maintain a "good" public family image. Moreover, the stigmatizing of actions works as a social control mechanism. It tells the stigmatized individual to hide or change his behavior in order to adhere to the standard (e.g., macho), while reaffirming the behavior of the source, the stigmatizer.

Rolando, who was born in the United States, also dealt with family rejection since early age because of what he calls his "sexuality." The rejection, he recalls, came in the form of distancing, mainly from his father. According to Rolando, he did not become fully aware of his father's distancing until a recent reflection on his life:

> My parents worked most of their lives. We'd see each other only at breakfast or dinner. We were good most of the time. In doing some self-analysis and talking with friends, [I realize now that] my dad and I didn't get along very well. My dad was kind of distant. I think because of my sexuality or what he perceived I was at early age. It's something that didn't dawn on me, or I thought it didn't affect or bother me, until probably in my early twenties.

The process that Rolando describes shows that the labeling of actions as unjust or discriminatory involves the acquisition of a language and understanding of oneself as a gay person. Now that he is openly gay and has socialized with peers and gay groups, he can attribute his father's actions to his homosexuality (and perhaps to his father's own negative attitudes toward homosexuality).

Rolando's predilection for dancing triggered the father's separation, stemming from the fact that dancing and dancing lessons in particular are not typical activities for a boy. It is an activity for girls. As Rolando articulates, dancing does not fit the cultural archetype of "macho":

> You don't hear me talking about my dad very much because, again, he was there, but he wasn't there. I guess he identified who I was at early age. He was the first to know with regards to gay and bisexual tendencies or sexual behavior. To put it straight, he abandoned me indirectly, subtly. What I know is that in his eyes, he didn't accept it and he kind of distanced. I was his favorite. And when he discovered . . . he just changed towards me. It didn't bother me at first

because I had my mom. . . . Now in retrospect, I see how he treated me. Now I can say that he was at a distance and it was the machismo, where the dancing isn't manly. The dancing kind of opened it. He said, "Wait, young boys don't get into that."

In his father's view, Rolando failed to fulfill the expectation of being a man, a macho. For the father, this could have meant disappointment and the loss of the bond between father and son. His father's initial rejection eventually grew into rejection by everybody in the family save for his mother. "My mom was there for everything," Rolando says. "She was very supportive. I brought her to some of my shows because she loved to dance too." When Rolando was in his early twenties, his mother became ill. Rolando took care of her for six years, despite the rejection he felt from his father and siblings. When his mother died, Rolando did not feel any obligation to stay and decided to leave. "Now, OK, I did my job. You guys don't accept me, don't want me around, what can I do?"

Another activist, Jack, says of his relationship with his father, "I was a very scared and timid child. I was constantly afraid. My father was very abusive." Jack recounts that his father yelled at him and beat him because he was not "rough" like other boys and was too close to his mother and sister. Actually, he relied on his mother and sister for solace. When Jack was in his teenage years, his parents divorced. Remarkably, now that Jack is thirty-six years old, the relationship with his father has improved. In the last five years, they started talking after several years of almost no communication. The father knows Jack is HIV positive, asks about Jack's boyfriend, and has gone to a couple of AIDS Walks with his son. Unlike many men, Jack's feelings of rejection by his father for not being "rough" have been assuaged.

Male figures, such as father and brothers, emerge in the lives of these GBTs as significant sources of stigma. This could be attributed to several factors. One is that men, as fathers, are expected to socialize their sons into male roles. Fathers may feel disappointed or failed by what they perceive as "unmanly" behavior of their sons—hence, they react negatively. Fathers and brothers may also feel threatened by the "unmanly" outlook of their sons or brothers. The womanlike behavior that they perceive in their sons or brothers poses the possibility that they may also act in that way, thereby undermining their maleness. Fathers' and brothers' masculinity may also be questioned by outsiders, who see them as "the father of the gay boy."

Mothers and sisters are also sources of stigmatization. In contrast to the male figures, their stigmatization is not as harsh (except for the case of transexual and drag-queen activists). Mothers frequently play the role of the supporter or comforter. Accordingly, mothers are watchful of their sons' behavior and make attempts to correct it if they see it as "unmanly" or "effeminate." Their reaction rarely involves physical mistreatment. Mateo's experience underscores this pattern. He describes his behavior as a ten-year-old boy as "very effeminate." His mother would correct his walking. "Don't walk like that—stand straight, walk straight," she warned. His aunts, however, were constantly criticizing his conduct. Mateo attributes this to the fact that they were overly devout Catholics, with a strict regard for gender roles and expectations. Mateo himself participated in the Roman Catholic youth movement in Mexico and had sex with the priest leader of his group:

> My behavior, especially my manners, was very effeminate. It was the typical behavior of a homosexual person. I'd sit delicately. I was fussy when eating. I recall my aunts telling me, "Don't sit that way. Don't cross your legs. Don't suck your finger. Don't walk that way. Don't talk like that."

Originally from Brazil, Ramiro goes further and describes his mother as "homophobic," despite having a gay man as her best friend:

> I remember my mother loving this friend, but somehow I think my mother knew I was gay and she was very worried about it. "Don't cross your legs." And she'd slap me and say, "Boys don't do that." . . . I remember going to buy a bicycle. Boys had bicycles that had a bar in the middle. I wanted a girl's bike, because I thought it'd be easier to get in and out. Of course, she thought it was a sign of my homosexuality. She was very homophobic.

This is not to minimize the stigma that mothers and sisters attach to homosexuality or gender nonconformity. Labeling a behavior as "feminine" and subsequently correcting a behavior because it is not "boylike" may harm a boy's image and relationships with his family, as it will be seen later in this chapter, in the same way as physical mistreatment can. To be called a "girl" could be construed by a boy to mean that he is weak, temperamental, and passive. In addition, such derogatory name-calling suggests deviance because one's behavior is in conflict with the expectations of peers (e.g., brothers and other boys).

If gender transgressing behavior and thoughts were measured by some objective standard, sexual relations between persons of the same sex, cross-dressing, and transgender identity may be considered as extremes on the spectrum. For that reason, they would be subject to the most severe forms of stigmatization. As suggested in Salvador's story, it is not uncommon to find accounts of sexual encounters among young siblings or cousins of the same sex. Similarly, it is not uncommon to find family members punishing such behaviors. For instance, Alfonso, who is HIV positive, got scolded

and beaten, along with his cousin, when they were found in the bathroom
touching each other:

> The first sexual experience, that I can recall, was with my cousin. We were about
> ten or eleven years old. We locked ourselves in the bathroom one time [when]
> we were visiting them. Our families thought we were out in the streets. Then,
> they found us. "What are you doing?" "Nothing," I said. But my cousin said
> we were touching each other. He got punished and beaten. I got reprimanded.

Within the family sphere and during childhood, drag queens and transexuals (male to female) invariably report the most severe stigma. The life stories
show that this may be due to the fact that from an early age their behavior
conflicted with others' expectations of their assigned gender. Furthermore,
in the eyes of the family, their behavior was evident, open, and persistent.
Ruby said, "I was born with mannerisms." *Mannerism* is frequently used
as a euphemism for feminine behavior. The behavior of these children (now
drag queens, transgenders, and transexuals) clearly crossed gender boundaries and could not be easily concealed. Ruby's childhood is illustrative of the
physical and verbal abuse experienced by this subgroup of *compañeros*. As
a child in Puerto Rico, she was beaten, rejected, and secluded by her mother
and stepfather. Her biological father had gone to California to live his life
as a gay man:

> Sincerely, I didn't have a childhood . . . I was born with mannerisms. I remember
> in Puerto Rico, they called me *pato* since I was in fifth grade. . . . *Pato* is like
> saying *faggot* or *maricón*. My mom would cover my head when we'd go out. She
> didn't want me to have male friends, because I wouldn't stop talking about
> them, she'd say. If I hung with the girls, she'd say that I'd learn girly ways. So
> she wouldn't let me go out. At 8 o'clock, go to school and at 3:30, come home
> directly, to clean, sweep floors, and wash clothes. I'd bring home Barbie from
> a neighbor's home. If I was caught by my mom, I'd get punished. She'd put me
> kneeling on rice for an hour, or hit me with a ruler. My stepfather was worse
> than Mom. He'd hit me with a whip so hard that you could see the marks in
> my body. He wanted me to act like a man.

Going to School

After family, school is the second most important gender socialization site
in the lives of Latino GBTs. School creates and reproduces social construc-
tions of femininity and masculinity through several mechanisms (Chodorow
1978). One is the separation of spaces and activities by sex. For instance,
boys and girls may be seated apart in the classroom. They may be divided
to receive information on sexuality and reproduction. Oftentimes, boys and

girls are also put in separate sports and teams. Another mechanism involves the content of the instruction in subjects such as biology and history, which may portray males and females as having different and perhaps opposite roles and values in society. A third device by which children are further socialized into gender roles is their interactions with teachers and peers. Teachers, in a similar manner as parents, engage in modeling gendered conduct, while peers provide social norms and models. The stories of Latino GBTs make clear that implicit in the gender socialization taking place in school is the stigmatization of conduct and thoughts that cross gender boundaries.

Fabian, for instance, still speaks with anger about his schoolteacher in Mexico, who told the class that boys who have sex with other boys were a "hopeless case." At the time, Fabian was about ten years old and had been "playing" sexually with his cousins since the age of seven:

> One day, this teacher, a stinking woman . . . we were in biology, and she went on saying that a boy who has sex with another boy is a hopeless case. But she said it in a very derogatory way, like nothing can be done about it. So, I thought, I'm having sex with other boys; that means I'd be gay forever. At the moment I felt such anguish, I'd cry and cry. I got in a terrible crisis.

While Fabian's anger arises in part from this event, it finds its origin in a set of experiences that led him to what he calls an "emotional crisis" and later to a failed marriage with a woman. Now thirty-two and living an openly gay life in Chicago, he sees those early experiences (such as the teacher's comment) as efforts from others to undermine his sexuality, which only caused him distress.

Mateo had an experience similar to Fabian. Mateo says that his schoolteacher, a man, in Mexico put him on the soccer team in an effort to change his behavior:

> I hated soccer, but the teacher said, "You have to play soccer." Supposedly to change my behavior and my manners; to change me from homosexual to a normal boy. They wouldn't say it that way, but the facts said it. Facts speak more than words. It's understood.

Mateo's explanation once again highlights the existence of an implicit gender system that dictates the lives and subjective meanings (or self-images) of these men. In this system, the term *normal* suggests not being homosexual, having a masculine demeanor, and adhering to the established gender division of spaces and activities such as playing soccer. This system does not require the explicit nature of a spoken language—"Facts speak more than words."

Yet, Mateo was also called names in school. Name-calling along with mockery and rejection are the most common types of stigmatization in school, and their main sources are peers. As Mateo recounts, other boys in school (girls are rarely, if at all, mentioned) frequently label and make fun of boys whose manners are perceived as feminine:

> [In elementary school] the boys would notice my mannerisms. They were always calling me like *marica*. . . . It was very insulting and it'd upset me a lot. Then I changed schools. I thought that things would change, being in a new environment and around older kids. The insults and the *mariquitas* started again. Obviously I'd get very upset and cry.

Sometimes, the mockery and ridicule are not triggered by demeanor (e.g., mannerisms) exhibited by a boy in public. Rather, they are the result of rumors, which spread information about the private behavior of a boy and question his masculinity. Humberto, a forty-eight-year-old U.S. native, was the victim of such rumors in high school. While in junior high, Humberto was having sexual relations with a neighbor. Later, when Humberto and his neighbor were in high school, Humberto told him he was not interested in having sex with him anymore. This triggered the rumors:

> I went to him and told him that I had met a girl, and if he'd please just leave me alone. He did. But what he did was, he went back to the school and told everybody that I was queer. That I was sucking his dick and he was doing this to me and going on and stuff. The people would come to me and say, "Oh, you're so and so. You suck, how do you call it . . . dick, don't you?"

Humberto's story also addresses another issue concerning the gender and sexual system of which he is a part. Men who perform oral sex on other men—as opposed to receive oral sex—are the "queer," the ones being stigmatized. This aspect of the gender system in many Latin American countries has been noted by several scholars (Carrillo 2002; Díaz 1998; Prieur 1998; Parker 1991; Carrier 1995). Under this system, the penetrative sexual behavior (either oral or anal) is rarely stigmatized. Sometimes, it is understood as evidence of a boy's or a man's masculinity. By contrast, the recipient's behavior is often stigmatized with labels such as "queer."

Boys and teenagers who are perceived and labeled as "feminine" or with "mannerism," often experience isolation in school. This isolation is the result of the rejection by their peers, who do not want to be associated with them. Deeming the effeminate boys unfit for activities such as soccer, they are excluded by peers. The labeled boys perceive such rejection and may consciously withdraw from their peers. As George's experience in Mexico illustrates, they feel that they do not fit in with their peers' interests. Furthermore, they want to avoid the name-calling and mockery:

So, that's how I spent my junior high years, with insults. Many times they made me cry. Once, they made me cry so much, that I couldn't cry anymore. I covered my face with my arms, and I cried and cried. . . . They told me vulgarities, like faggot, whore, and such.

Sometimes, we'd go to museums and camps, and . . . I'd go my own way . . . I'd separate from them, because I couldn't be with the rest of the guys . . . they wouldn't let me. If I were close to them, they'd start calling me names.

In a few instances, stigmatization in school involves beating and sexual harassment. Boys and young men who are labeled as feminine are sometimes viewed as sex objects that desire sexual contact—even penetration. In a peculiar chain of events, Alfonso encountered physical abuse and sexual harassment on two different occasions in high school. First, a classmate who used to call him names hit Alfonso for no apparent reason. An acquaintance came to Alfonso's defense. He expected sex in return:

He didn't like me. He'd say I was *joto, maricón*. He hit and pushed me twice. He stopped when I told him I'd report him to the principal, which I did the following day. He got suspended for about a week. He was very angry at me when he got back. So this classmate, who was after me, told me he'd take care of him. We were leaving school, and the other guy started bothering me, so my classmate intervened and beat him up.

Then, this classmate wanted me to return the favor by having sex with him. We were at my house doing homework. He took his clothes off and asked me to touch him. I was hesitant. I touched him, but we didn't have sex. I was afraid of my family showing up. The bottom line is that he wanted to rape me. He grabbed me, forcing me. But I didn't let him. We struggled.

This incident took place years after Alfonso and his cousin were caught in the bathroom touching each other naked. Then, he was scolded by his parents.

The stigma that *compañeros* faced as children and youths in school puts them in even more vulnerable positions. The name-calling, mockery, rejection, and beating that they endured were not isolated or single incidents. A few of them, like Alfonso, were able to fight back on a few occasions. Many, however, opted to remain silent to avoid further stigmatization.

Going to Therapy

Although homosexuality ceased to be considered a psychiatric disorder in 1973 in the United States, many psychologists and lay people still treat it as a condition or anomaly that needs to be cured. Of course, most GBTs are not institutionalized. In the following accounts, parents and the men themselves turn to psychological therapy either to modify the men's "feminine" behavior or to adjust the men's personality to their social environment. Fabian's parents, for instance, went to family therapy in order to determine what was troubling their young son, whose teacher had told him that boys who had sex with other boys were a "hopeless case"—an assertion that made Fabian cry:

> They'd seen my crying, but I didn't tell them why. We went to a psychologist for family therapy. There it eventually came up that I had had sex with other boys. Everybody was very understanding. "All boys play with other boys." We were in therapy for about two years. And things got better. I got out of the crisis. It was the beginning of my adolescence.

Later in his life, however, Fabian turned again to therapy. In his early twenties, he went to group therapy because he "didn't want to be gay." Fabian was in therapy for six years. Now, he looks at those years of therapy with anger and pain because the psychologist tried to change his homosexual feelings:

> I decided to go to therapy again. I went for six years because I didn't want to be gay. I wanted to be with girls. Actually, I'm very pissed at this therapist, because he's very biased. During my therapy, all the attention was focused on "What about girls?" He'd never explore my feelings about boys. "Do you like them?" "Why do you feel guilty about your feelings?"
>
> He'd ask people in the group: "So, do you think Fabian is gay?" Of course, everybody would say, "No, I don't think so." So it's like the support didn't help me. I was just so fucking pissed.

Fabian spent several years of his life in therapy. His parents initially sought the help of the psychologist to figure out what was troubling their son. In doing so, they likely socialized Fabian into psychological therapy. Fabian learned to see psychological therapy as a mechanism to deal with life's troubles. So, Fabian began to see his homosexual desire as a problem and as within the framework of psychology. The therapy that he attended later as a young adult clearly exacerbated the conflict Fabian was experiencing between his homosexual desires and his gender role as a man. The psychologist posed heterosexual identity as the only viable path.

Andres, who is fifty-three years old and a generation older than Fabian, was sent to therapy by a schoolteacher. In high school, at age fifteen, Andres had two close friends. Their schoolmates used to call them "the three Maries." One of them was caught having sex beneath the stairwell. The three friends were subsequently sent to a psychologist.

Parents and teachers are the main socializing agents in these men's childhoods. They are also primary sources of stigma. Parents and teachers seek out other sources such as psychology in order to deal with their own anxieties created by the "feminine" conduct of the children. These sources (in this case, psychology and its practitioners), then, become socializing agents and authorities for the children. Regardless of whether the psychological therapy is seen as negative, overtly stigmatizing, or helpful, psychology becomes a dominant framework for the children to later define and deal with their sexuality.

Alfonso, for example, decided to consult a psychologist during college, when he became conflicted about his sexual relations with other men:

> When I was 21, I decided to seek professional help with a psychologist from the university services. This doctor was old, about 60 or 65. He told me, "You can't be homosexual. Your role as a human being is to establish a family, to get married and have children. That's nature's law."

Psychological therapy may actually be a source of stigma when it denies the existence of homosexuality as a valid life option, making it an abnormality and privileging heterosexual identity and sexual behavior. In addition, it stigmatizes when it defines an individual's sexual behavior as a problem, or as a problem located in that individual's psyche. As adults, it is not uncommon for these GBTs to continue seeking psychological therapy to deal with their lives' tribulations, including homosexuality.

Police Harassment

When asked why he came to the United States, Marc says that in his native Peru, "I had problems with the police. They beat me because I was gay." Marc explains that even though he did not always appear gay, just seeing him with other men or knowing that he was not married seemed sufficient justification for police to abuse him:

> Once the police attacked me only because they saw me chatting with a friend. We had left *un bar de ambiente* [a gay bar] about 8 at night, and we sat down to chat. The police arrested us and took us to a close-by building. They beat us. They told us we were homosexuals. We told them we weren't. But they thought we were, because we told them we weren't married. They punched us in the stomach. Then, they asked us if we had any money. We gave them all we had with us so that they would let us go.

When these *compañeros* begin exploring their social and homosexual lives outside family and school, they become the targets of other sources of stigma, such as police forces. Regardless of whether homosexual behavior is prohibited or regulated by law, police abuses toward GBT persons take place (now with less frequency) in both Latin American countries and the United States. Police personnel (men, in most instances) operate as members of society and act in accordance with society's gender system, stigmatizing men whose behavior crosses gender roles. Thus, they likely see GBTs as criminals, lumping them together with drug users and sex workers and even deserving of violence and abuse. Police stigmatization of GBTs includes raids on bars or private homes, arrest, physical and verbal violence, and bribery. Mateo's experiences in Guadalajara, Mexico, offer a glimpse into the stigma among police. He, like Marc, ultimately left his home country searching for a place free of this abuse:

> We were in this gay bar, when all of a sudden one night two or three police cars arrived. They ran all over us. Denying our rights, they put us against the walls, as if we were criminals. They searched us for drugs. They videotaped us and took us to the police station. We put all our money together to pay the fine, but we couldn't pay for everybody. So, six of us stayed in.
>
> We were let free the following day. I was 36 hours in jail. And the policemen, with their nepotism and arrogance, think that because you're gay they have the right to mistreat you, beat you, humiliate you, and to step on your dignity. It also happened to me once in Mexico City. There I confronted a police man. "The fact that I'm gay doesn't give you the right to get into my private life. My life is not your business." The guy insisted on asking if I was prostituting.
>
> The incident in Guadalajara was different, because there were a lot of transvestites. Many of the transvestite boys would prostitute. *Pagan justos por pecadores* [the just pays for the sinner]. The police put you in the same boat. They think you're depraved, selling drugs and your body, that you're the worst of society.

As implied by Mateo, police and gay men see transvestites, or drag queens, as easier and more deserving targets of mistreatment than gay men. The transgression of gender boundaries is more flagrant among transvestites, drag queens, and transsexual persons than gay men. Thus, they experience more frequent and harsher abuse from police than do gay men. For instance, Gustavo, a fifty-one-year-old who also goes by the name of Carmen when dressed as a woman, says that he was beaten and jailed on several occasions while living in Mexico City:

> I began dressing as a woman when I was 20-something years old. But in Mexico . . . Even if one is not dressed as a woman, if one walks wiggling, a little queeny, the police come and get you. The times I have been jailed, have all been in Mexico, not here [in the United States]. And it's been because of being gay, no other reason.
>
> Once it happened after a drag-queen contest, which I won in Mexico City. I was very elegant and wearing a tremendous wig. We had finished the contest, and a woman friend asked me to walk with her to make a phone call by the

corner. She was my ride, so I agreed to join her. While she was on the phone, I waited outside the booth. Then the *judiciales* [federal police] come and force me in the car. It wasn't a police car, it was like an undercover car.

My friend yelled, "What's going on? Where are you taking my sister?" One of the guys replied, "What sister?—this is a faggot!" So, there I was all dressed up and only with a small velvet purse. I had no I.D. cards and almost no money with me. The police started driving me around. One of the guys pulled my wig off. Then the other guy wanted to take my nails off, because he thought they were false. He wanted to pull them out. It was horrible and still hurts just talking about it. Then they took the little money I had, my rings, my earrings, everything. "You get out of here, faggot! Son of the bitch! If you turn around we'll shoot you!"

Gustavo eventually took a taxi to his home, where his worried friend was waiting.

Dislocation

We learned from Marc and Mateo that the stigma experienced by GBTs sometimes leads to leaving their native countries. Before coming to the United States, Marc moved from Lima to a smaller town, hoping people would be more warm and friendly than in the city. Unfortunately, he found himself again facing questions about being single and not having a girlfriend, and with almost no "lugares de ambiente" (gay places) where he could socialize with other gay men. He returned to Lima, saved some money and migrated to the United States. "I faced so much discrimination, so many problems for being gay," he explains. "It was a lot of pressure in Peru. I felt forced to leave and come here." Mateo reached the same conclusion but took a different route. After his arrest in Guadalajara, Mateo went to Canada and applied for refugee status. His application was denied. Mateo is now in the process of appealing that decision.

Men from Latin America are compelled to leave their birth countries to escape from the name-calling, harassment, and the potential stigma they bring into their families. Perhaps Vladimir best described the flight when he said that he left his homeland "to live my gay life in freedom, without prejudice." Men from Latin America who have migrated to the United States, including Vladimir, see the latter as the most viable alternative to their own countries.

> I came here [from Mexico] to live my life . . . to live my private life with freedom. I feel liberated. I can be who I am without the fear of been pointed out, without worrying about what others would say. The culture from which one comes marginalizes you. There is such a pressure, that you have [to] live a double life.

. . . It's very conflicting to live two lives. You get tangled here and disentangled there, always trying to hide, to put on a mask and hide your own identity.

Oftentimes, migrating to another country involves a sense of rejection from family. Men like Vladimir feel that their families and the larger society have rejected them. Dislocation, thus, becomes an outcome of stigma.

Thalia, a self-identified transgender, migrated to San Francisco after her mother threw her out of the house in Mexico City. Now, at the age of nineteen, Thalia feels rejected by her family and school peers in Mexico. She recounts her tortuous journey to San Francisco—a trip that she made with the aid of a coyote.

My dad died of cancer when I was 11, but he never bothered me. But my mom did notice what was going [on] with me. "You better watch your mannerisms," she'd warn me. . . . Growing up was horrible because I didn't have the freedom to express myself. In the school, I was always the *mariconcito*. I used to have my hair to my shoulders, so they'd call me gay.

At age 14 I left home. [My mom] said I was the shame of the family. It really bothered me, so I left the house and went to Saltillo. I spent several days there and took a freight train to Monterrey. There I made some money helping a woman selling tacos in the bus station. I took a bus to Nuevo Laredo, where I lived for several months until I got some money to pay the coyote to cross me.

Marta's story has striking similarities to Thalia's. Marta is a fifty-four-year-old from Puerto Rico who has lived most of her adult life in Chicago. Growing up, she endured the abuse of her mother because of her womanlike conduct. At age fourteen, her mother found her in bed with a boyfriend and asked Marta to leave the house:

My boyfriend and I went to a birthday party. I was wearing a nice dress and high heels. That night I was home alone, so when we got back from the party, I went to bed all dressed. In the morning, when my mom got in, she asked, "What are you doing here?" Then she went to my room and punched me. She kicked him out and told me, "You're out of here." Rushing, I got a pillowcase and took all I could, some clothes and things like that.

Then I went to school. Of course, I couldn't stop crying. My friend Rita saw me and I told her what had happened. "My mom kicked me out of the house because of this."

My mom had never seen me in woman's clothes. She'd heard, but had never seen me. "Come to my house," she [Rita] offered me. So, she talked with her mother and they let me stay with them.

Ariel was also thrown out of the house by his mother. His situation is different, however, because of his family's association with Jehovah's Witnesses.

Ariel was a church elder at the age of twenty-two, but he was aware of his homosexual desires as a teenager. "Once I overdid my feminine manners and all the family's males and my stepfather gave me a speech." He stepped down from his position in the church in an effort to come to terms with his homosexuality and returned home to live with his family in the Chicago suburbs:

> From one of my trips to the city, I had brought the *Windy City Times* [a local gay newspaper]. I put it under the bed. That Sunday, I went to the Gay Pride Parade. When I came back, I found the newspaper spread all over my bed. I knew who had done it. We had the talk and she told me, "You have to leave the house and forget that you have a mother."

The moment of departure from family and country define the lives of many of these Latino activists. Having been expelled, they have to create their own new lives, including a new "familia." Ariel said:

> I began to reconstruct my life, to learn who I am, to learn to live on my own, and to learn to be honest with myself and to others. I met new friends, good friends who have come to be like my family.

Dislocation and displacement give rise to the adoption of a public identity as a gay man or transgender person and the socialization with other gay or transgender persons (topics that will be covered in chapters 4 and 7). This makes dislocation one of the most significant experiences.

Internalization

The internalization of stigma related to gender nonconformity, frequently referred to as internalized homophobia, is the adoption of others' negative views to define the self. Internalization takes place when a GBT person, or a person with homosexual desires, embraces the predominant negative societal views toward nonconforming gender behaviors to define him or herself and others. Internalized homophobia is difficult to assess empirically, and frequently it is treated as an unproblematic concept in psychology and public health literature. The problem lies in that the concept assumes both positive and negative definitions of the self, which, in turn, assume the existence of a standard. In this case, the norm has been the definition of "gay" established by white middle-class groups in North America and Western Europe (Chauncey 1994). Embracing a public identity as a gay man is seen as the positive definition of the self. Thus, homosexual individuals, or those who do not conform to that standard, are said to have internalized homophobia (a negative definition of the self). It could be the case, but it is also possible (and I believe true) that there are many forms of expressing and living homosexual desires that do not lead to a negative view of the self.

Another problematic assumption is the unchanging nature of internalization. The phenomenon is not a personality trait. It is a framework learned as a part of the early socialization process, which could be discarded when proven to be incorrect. It can be completely dismissed as a tool to see the self and the world, or it can be used discriminately.

With that view of internalized stigma, the life histories of *compañeros* reveal relatively little internalized homophobia. They show that its presence was limited, for the most part, to short time periods, and that when not used to define the self, it is deployed to see and judge others (e.g., transgender people). In addition, the life stories make it clear that internalization causes personal distress.

Eliezer's case stands out from the others because he is still very much conflicted about his sexual orientation. This conflict is confounded by what he describes as an eating problem that he developed during childhood:

> I know that if I don't confront my problems right now, it's going to be more difficult later, because of my long-term problem with food. It has always been like an addiction. It has a lot to do with childhood, because I grew up with an alcoholic father. He found an escape in alcohol; I found it in food.
>
> I think my biggest problem is my identity as a homosexual man. I can't get to accept myself. In college, I had some gay friends, but there was a part of me that I couldn't accept. Even now living here in San Francisco, it's like who you are has nothing to do with the place where you are. Sometimes one thinks that living in San Francisco is the best, but I think it has more to do with oneself, as a person, and with how one grew up. My dad abused me, emotionally and physically, because I think he perceived my homosexuality. He yelled a lot at me and wanted me to be like *machito*. So I think I used food to rebel against him. I ate as a way of revenge. But then I realized that I'm the only one getting hurt by it. I'm angry at my dad because of all the problems I have now.

Clearly, Eliezer has done some self-reflection in order to come to a better understanding of himself as a gay. He is twenty-nine years old and has a degree in psychology from his native Mexico. Eliezer explains how his education and training have helped him understand what he is going through. He still cannot implement the changes that he thinks are needed to address his homosexuality:

> I don't believe my problem has much to do with losing weight, as with dealing with my emotional issues about homosexuality. I'm very angry about being homosexual. I envy my heterosexual friends, because I grew up with the Catholic dream of getting married at some point in my life. I don't necessary like the

idea of being with a woman, but I enjoy the idea of preparing our wedding, choosing her wedding dress, and riding a limousine to a pretty Catholic church; a Mexican-style church.

Echoing the predominant lay and religious ideals, Eliezer views marriage with a woman (not with a man) as the norm, the symbol of one's realization, and perhaps as the only route to a fulfilling life. As a gay man, he knows that he cannot marry. In following his logic, he arrives at the conclusion that something is wrong with him, not with the idea of marriage. In addition, it can be deduced from this narrative that one of the sources of Eliezer's negative view of himself, or internalized stigma, is his Catholic upbringing, which has been reinforced by his father's stigmatizing actions and Eliezer's eating disorder.

Another aspect Eliezer is grappling with is the meaning of the word *homosexual* (in its Spanish and English usages). As he explains, he avoids using the word because of the negative portrayals of homosexuals in the media, especially in Mexico. To some extent, he seems to endorse those negative views, underscoring the conflict between his homosexual behavior and society's expectations:

> Honestly, I dislike the word *homosexual*. I prefer the word gay because it's gentler. The word *homosexual* means like criminal, as the newspapers in Mexico use it to describe us. A newspaper never says, "A heterosexual killed in an accident," but of course they say, "A homosexual killed." *Homosexual* represents a part of me that I don't like.

As he continues, Eliezer notes that he prefers the word *gay* to describe himself, both in Mexico and the United States. In his rationale, it is evident that he is uncomfortable with the meaning of the word homosexual with which he became acquainted in Mexico. Its meaning is different from the meaning he attaches to the word *gay*:

> The word *gay* is easier. It represents another social class. It represents different contexts, Mexico and United States. I feel like it comes from a different class, from college-educated people, or from the Castro. It's like the word *queer*. *Queer* is a bit better . . . I use the word *gay* more when I speak English and also when speaking Spanish. I use it so people know that I come from another [higher] social status or educational level.

Eliezer's comparison reveals his understanding of two different social contexts, from which different conceptualizations of homosexuality emerge. In Mexico, Eliezer learned that *homosexual* connotes elements of anomaly and criminality. By contrast, for Eliezer, *gay* connotes a degree of education, social status, and whiteness. These are meanings of *gay* that Eliezer has learned in San Francisco. They are the meanings that he wants to portray.

Having been raised in Mexico, Eliezer sees homosexual persons in a negative light. In a move to try to come to terms with his own homosexuality,
he has tried to take on the word *gay,* which offers him a positive meaning
while distancing him from what he perceives as the "Mexican homosexual."

Unlike Eliezer, most of the other activists and volunteers expressed internalized homophobia as occurring in the past and for a limited time period.
Victor, who was ridiculed and called "faggot" as a child in Chicago, says
he "grew to hate that feminine side" of himself. Now at the age of twenty-
three, Victor says he is "more comfortable" with himself:

> When I was ridiculed, I tried to prove that I wasn't like that. "Oh I'm not
> feminine. I'm not feminine." I grew to hate it. As a child, I'd feel like: "I don't
> like that part of me."
>
> Everything, the repressing and ridiculing built up. It was very hard for me,
> because you have the religious part of it, together with the family and the com-
> munity. Mexican men have to be machos. I was always made fun of. That's
> why it took me so long to accept myself. There were many times when I'd go
> to bed to crying. I pleaded to God: "God, I don't want to be this way. Please,
> make a miracle. Please, change me. I don't want my family to go through this.
> I don't want people to make fun of me the rest of my life."

Victor's internalization of homosexual stigma is expressed as a "hate" toward himself or a dislike of himself because he is attracted to other men.
This internalization is the outcome of being called names and made fun of
as a child because of what he calls "mannerisms." It is also the outcome
of Catholicism, the family, and other social institutions that reproduce or
sustain gender constructs (e.g., men are machos). As children, they learn at
home, school, playgrounds, churches, and through media that their attraction toward other boys and their conduct, labeled feminine, is abnormal
and flawed.

There are two reasons why there is, relatively speaking, little internalized homophobia among these activists. First, the majority of them have
adopted a public gay or transgender identity, which implies that, for the
most part, they have unlearned some of the internalized stigma. Second,
they are volunteers and activists in LGBT and HIV/AIDS organizations.
As I address in chapter 7, this involvement has helped them readdress the
stigma so that they attribute it not to character flaw but to society's negative
attitudes toward homosexual and transgender persons (Ramirez-Valles et
al. 2005). I discuss these two explanations in chapters 6 and 7.

Yet another form in which internalized stigma is expressed among this
group of Latino gay men is in their negative views toward transgender
persons and drag queens. This may also be characterized as a community

or group level internalized stigma. Angelica labeled this form as *misogyny*—that is, an aversion toward women. Angelica, who is twenty-six years old, recently experienced this form of stigmatization when she was fired from a health club in San Francisco:

> It was discrimination because I was a queen. They have gay people working there, but they are like the Ken-doll types of gay guys. Misogyny and internalized homophobia are the root for gay men not to like queens. Queens could make gay men question themselves. Gay guys have to prove that they are men because they have been called faggots, and faggots are not men.

Marta's view concurs with Angelica's. Marta also felt discriminated against in the AIDS organization where she works because she was transgender. The organization had a position open at a level higher than Marta's, but she was not asked to interview or even to apply. "Only because of my physical appearance. They wouldn't give me the opportunity because of the way I look, and it's worse in the gay community." Marta has experienced rejection in different situations from the gay male population, especially Latino gay males. She attributes this to gay men's fears of being labeled "feminine," though some gay men would like to have the freedom to dress and act like a woman:

> The majority of gay males can't stand being next to a drag queen. However, on Halloween, you go to any disco and you can see them in drag. One reason is that their family, culture, and religion don't allow them. They'd allow him [a drag queen] to be out of the closet, but they tell him, "We allow you, but don't come with your little faggot things."
>
> We have realized something that gay guys can't. We are giving a look that they can't, or don't allow themselves to have. I have the freedom to do it and that makes them uncomfortable.

Angelica's and Marta's narratives speak of the internalized dominant gender constructs among men in the gay community. While many gay men have contended with gender constructs, they use the same constructs in relation to drag queens and transgender persons. This suggests a slight revision in the internalized (and prevailing) gender constructs, by which a gay or homosexual category or identity can exist as long as they do not transgress the categories of male and female. Thus, a gay male can accept himself and others alike to the extent that he keeps his outlook within the parameters of masculinity.

The Negative Consequences of Stigma

The accounts by these *compañeros* have already given us a glance at how stigma has negatively affected their lives. The name-calling, ridicule, beating and rejection from family, peers, school, religion, and media, along with the resulting dislocation and internalization, have caused them short- and long-term negative effects, such as dropping out of school, financial strain, isolation, distress, low self-esteem, depression, and suicidal ideation.

"I had suffered a lot," Simon says as he looks at his life, which has run its course from a wealthy upbringing in Central America to a life with HIV in San Francisco at the age of sixty-three. Simon was verbally abused by his mother and harassed while in school in the United States because he was "a little effeminate." He explains "that didn't hurt me psychologically." The stigma hurt materially, however, in that it eliminated certain life opportunities:

> I never got the jobs I'd have liked, because of my mother. I wanted to study art and interior decorating. My mother told me I couldn't do that because it was for "weird people . . ." If I wouldn't have been gay, I'd have married a wealthy woman from Nicaragua. I'd be a millionaire, with five children, and a nice home. I'm not bitter. I had no choice, but I could have had all of that.

If Simon had not been "effeminate," his family's business and wealth would most likely have been passed on to him. He would have subsequently stayed in his native Nicaragua. This is because a cultural gender script and actual state regulations expect heterosexual individuals (specifically, married men) to reproduce capital or wealth. Simon provides an example of how gay men and nongay men have different degrees of access to financial and social capital. Stigma negatively affects many GBTs in their access to education, money, and family and social network resources.

Emotional distress, nonetheless, is the most commonly found outcome in this sample of Latinos. This is manifested in emotional crisis, depression, low self-esteem, or thoughts about suicide. Ariel went through a very difficult time when the conflict between his religious values (Jehovah's Witnesses) and homosexual desires intensified:

> I lived like that [with the conflict] until I was 22 years old. There was a conflict between the person I knew I was and the person I projected as a minister. It was causing me lots of emotional and psychological trauma. Even more because my church condemned homosexuality. It was very upsetting to have to go up to the platform every Sunday, to speak against homosexuality and morality, knowing who I was inside. Back then I got very depressed.

Ariel's conflict deepened because he fell in love and started a sexual relationship with his roommate. The sexual relationship was on and off for several years. The feelings of guilt and of unrequited love led Ariel to three suicide attempts:

At that time, I tried to kill myself three times. I survived because of a miracle. Once I crashed my car. It was during a snow storm and I crashed the car against a concrete wall. I was bleeding when an elderly couple found me and took me to the hospital. I was getting more and more depressed and losing my position in the church. I left the church and moved to my parents' town. This guy followed me and we lived together again.

So the next time I tried to kill myself was at home. I waited for him to leave for work. I took many pills. He left work early and found me on the floor. I ended up in the hospital and about six weeks in a psychiatric unit. It was the best thing that could have happened to me. Those six weeks were very difficult, with a lot of analysis of my religious ideas and my family relations.

After those six weeks I did about six months of therapy. It was a very hard time, but well rewarded, with lots of self-examination.

Another *compañero,* Omar, tried to kill himself on two occasions, when he felt he had nothing to live for. At the age of ten in Mexico, Omar was already having sex with other boys and was frequently called *joto, maricón,* and *puto* (whore). In his early twenties he went back to live with his parents because he felt afflicted by his homosexual behavior and persistent acne. There he tried to end his life:

> Those four years that I was at my parents, I'd think were the last thing I'd do. I tried to commit suicide twice. My parents wouldn't let me sleep by myself. So for me it was like I had lived all. I had had fun and boyfriends. It was like an end.

Omar changed and felt "motivated to move on" when his father fell ill. He felt he needed to help his family financially and emotionally. Similarly, Gabriel contemplated ending his life, but he lived under somewhat different circumstances in California. When Gabriel was a teenager, he was repeatedly asked, "Are you gay? Are you gay?" His brothers and school friends would call him "sissy, faggot, and slowpoke," in part because he disliked boys' sports. Thus, he found himself not feeling "normal" and unlike the rest of the boys. In college, he succumbed to the stigma he had endured:

> In college, I was not out until my junior year. I liked boys, but never acted upon my thoughts. . . . I went through a very critical sexuality crisis in my sophomore year, where I just absolutely hated myself. I had really low self-esteem. I was having migraines, had never had them [before]. I had a lot of roommate problems, and then I ended up living alone, because I couldn't stand roommates any more.
>
> So I got my own room and, then . . . then I was just like suicidal. . . . Because of the pressure of not being normal. The pressure of being an outcast, being gay. I didn't want to come to terms and I would cry talking to God, "Why did you make me this way if I'm not even accepted? Why can't I just be normal? Why can't I just have a girlfriend like my friends and my brother?

Facing Stigma

This group of activists has not been a passive recipient of stigma. Since an early age, many have developed and used several strategies to cope with and to change the stigma toward nonconforming gender behavior. I distinguish coping from changing strategies (Ensel and Lin 1991; Pearlin et al. 1981; Meyer 1995). The former implies dealing with the impact and consequences of stigmatization, such that its negative effects are nullified or attenuated. Changing addresses the sources of stigma, thus aiming at social change. Both the gay and the AIDS movements emerged as social-change strategies. These are not mutually exclusive approaches, as individuals and groups may be working toward changing sources of stigma while coping with the stigmatizing environment.

Of course, as activists and volunteers, many of these Latinos are engaged in a social-change strategy. Many of them are involved because they want to change the sources of stigma toward nonconforming behavior, Latinos, and people living with HIV and AIDS. Others participate in the organizations to cope with their own stigmatizing experiences. Given the significance of this strategy in confronting stigma, I discuss it in more detail when I explore community involvement (chapters 6 and 7). Here I focus on individual approaches outside of activism and volunteerism that they have taken to deal with stigma toward nonconforming behavior. I label them: going straight; don't ask, don't tell; and confrontation. These strategies tend to fall under coping mechanisms. There are some instances in which change was the aim, albeit at the individual level.

"Going straight" refers to the strategy of trying to act "macho," or hiding the "feminine mannerisms" from others to avoid being called names or being ridiculed. Ramiro, from Brazil, and Victor, from Chicago, opted for this approach when other boys in school would call them "faggot." Ramiro explains: "The way I dealt with it was sometimes being one of them. Like playing basketball, volleyball, and being tough with them." In the same manner, Victor notes: "I'd always try to be more macho kind. Like more athletic. To prove to them that I wasn't that girly or prissy." Later in their lives, some of these men take a similar approach when in a nongay environment. Omar says, "When I go to straight bars with friends or coworkers, I behave like a straight person. If I'm with straight friends, I try to act normal, not as a gay."

The most singular case is that of Mario, who at age twenty felt compelled to marry a woman in El Salvador to avoid stigmatization. Mario grew up in a deeply religious and very active Protestant family. Despite having some awareness of his homosexual desires, he felt pressured by his religious beliefs and church to get married:

> When I was 19, I understood and said to myself, "The church will never accept me as a gay." That's where I got the idea of getting married. The church issue was such a big problem for me, that even when I was married, I was labeled as a married gay man. It was something that nobody would say, but I'd feel it.

Rolando calls his way of dealing with his sexuality a "don't-ask-don't-tell" attitude. This approach refers to an unspoken understanding among family members to avoid discussion of each others' sexuality. Rolando's experience (as well as Mario's) is unique among this group of activists, but not necessarily among the larger gay population. Rolando recounts that he grew up in the United States hearing his parents' negative comments about homosexual men. Now, as a gay man, he prefers not to talk about his homosexuality with his parents. This way, he will not disappoint them. He will also avoid their potentially stigmatizing reaction:

> I didn't want to disappoint them. I didn't want to hurt them. Not that I was ashamed of who I am. It's just that they have a different outlook. My parents think gay, bisexual people are wrong. I grew up with an attitude don't ask, don't tell. It's the way I've learned.
>
> My sexuality is my business. You see me as a person. It's not that I'm closeted, or holding back, or ashamed. No, I'm not, that's not important. It's what you are inside as a person.

Don't ask, don't tell and going straight work as coping mechanisms. As strategies, they do not aim at changing the source of stigma; instead, they diminish or suppress its expression and negative impact on the recipient. In contrast, the third and last strategy, confrontation, is aimed at the source of stigma. Confrontation involves efforts to dispute the source's claims, to silence and possibly to change the source's view of homosexuality at the individual level. Jimmy, for example, confronted his restaurant manager after he called Jimmy *pato* (faggot) in front of other people:

> [At first] I didn't say anything. I said, "OK, that's OK." But I couldn't focus on my job, I wanted to hide. He said it with such anger. I wait for the end of the day.
>
> Then I got him. "I want to speak with you," I asked him. "I know you're the manager and that you're in charge of everything here, but that doesn't give you the right to call me names, let alone in front of others," I said. "There are many people who understand that word. If you have a problem with me, so tell me." So he said, "I'm sorry. I'm sorry." I told him that "sorry" wasn't enough, because he had hurt my feelings.

When he was a child, Gustavo confronted boys who would call him names. At times, he even resorted to throwing punches. He stopped when his tactic backfired:

> In school there was always somebody who'd show me his erect penis underneath the desk, and someone who'd call me *maricón*. I'd get angry and hit them. We'd fight and I'd always win. Even by the house, once a kid called me *maricón* and I punched him.
>
> Later, his mother complained to my dad. I got the worst. My dad beat me, because I beat the other kid. From then on, when I'd hear "maricón," I'd lower my head and turn around.

Stigma toward nonconforming behavior is the process of labeling and discrediting individuals because they do not conform to the socially constructed ideas of man and woman. These activists are labeled, since early age, as abnormal, weird, sissy, *joto,* and *pato* among other derogatory terms because their actions, ideas, gestures, games, and friendships do not match the social expectations of a man or, as they usually referred to, a *macho.* Most of the stigmatization takes place in childhood and teenage years, and comes from family, school, peers, religion, and media.

The stigma takes the form of name-calling, verbal and physical abuse, ridiculing, harassing, rejection, distancing, and dislocation. Some of these *compañeros* come to perceive the world, or their society, as a place in which they are not welcome. They come to see themselves through the eyes of their oppressors, the stigmatizers, as stigma is internalized. That is when stigma triggers its most harmful effects, such as isolation, depression, and suicide. Regardless of its internalization, stigma frequently leads to material and nonmaterial adversity, some of which spans over a lifetime. Yet, internalization among these Latinos is, for the most part, transitory. They have fought, and continue to fight, internalization. One way in which they have done it, I argue through this book, is through their activism and volunteerism. The stigma they experience and perceive has led many of them to get involved in groups and organizations dealing with gay, Latino, and HIV/AIDS issues. Through this involvement they learn from peers and organizations to attribute the stigma not to themselves, but to others' (e.g., family, school, religion) negative views of behavior and thoughts that do not conform to the dominant gender roles.

CHAPTER THREE

THE MEANINGS OF LATINO

The word *Latino* means nothing and everything. It can be an empty category. It can also be full of meanings and contradictions. *Latino* is a socially constructed concept or category when referring to a group. Its existence and meanings are contingent on a particular social and historical context. In this instance, the context is the U.S. racial system. Outside the United States, *Latino* is almost nonexistent. If it does exist, its meanings are different and perhaps less powerful than those in the United States. To think of *Latino* as a social construct is not to deny the actual consequences of its use on the individuals categorized as such. One of the most significant consequences is the stigma and the discriminatory practices exercised upon those people referred to as Latinos.

In the United States, we use *Latino* as a label to categorize people as a race, ethnic group, or minority. As Michel Foucault proposed (1976/1990), labels such as this one are created to manage populations. One of the features of power is to create and name the other (e.g., people not defined as white and thought of as different) through such labels. In doing so, it reduces human complexity to a set of characteristics or a stereotype, which then become an identity. The creation of this Latino identity, however, cannot be attributed solely to what is usually thought of as the sites of power, namely, state institutions and the mostly white male ruling group. Individuals and groups categorized as Latinos have also been active participants in the creation and maintenance of such identity (Skerry 1993).

The term *Latino* contains some ambiguity. Both lay people and state institutions (e.g., census) frequently equate *Latino* with race, ethnicity, or minority status (Skerry 1993). Its use is not empty when we see the enormous variation of so-called races included in the Latino category. But, it becomes devoid of meaning when we think of race as a social construct. Race does not exist as a homogeneous group of people sharing either a particular set of genes or physiological features (Wilkinson and King 1987; Cooper and David 1986). Races, like "black" and "white," are merely the product of social factors in the context of power relations and in a given historical period. In the United States, race has been created through state regulations such as segregated schooling and housing programs, and through daily life practices such as attitudes, harassment, and verbal abuse (Roediger 1991; Wolpe 1986; Anthias 1990).

Latinos can not be thought of as an ethnic group. An ethnic group refers to a group (or groups) of people who share a culture, that is, language, religion, food, music, and a structure of relations among individuals (e.g., marriage, family). Hence, to think of *Latino* as an ethnicity is to echo the dominant racial discourse. As the life histories of *compañeros* attest, individuals referred to as Latinos come from a variety of cultural milieus: residential projects in Southern California farms; a small town in Cuba; southern Brazil; the Bronx in New York City; the Mexico–United States border; Tierra Amarilla, New Mexico; a Native American reservation in Colorado; the Pilsen neighborhood in Chicago; Morelia, Michoacán; the outskirts of Mexico City; and Nicaragua.

Although not comprising an ethnic group, Latinos could be thought of as a minority group. Here, I refer to *minority group* not in terms of numeric denotation, but in the oppressed sense of the word (Skerry 1993). That is, Latinos can be considered members of an oppressed group based on their position in power relations. The dominant discourse frequently treats them as such, as in the case of welfare programs and affirmative action policies. Those programs and policies, however, reproduce constructs of race and power relationships (e.g., between those called *Latinos* and *whites*) more than alleviate or change power differences.

In the understanding of Latino as a minority group lies the potential for collective action and social change. When a group of Latinos as diverse as the group of activists represented in this book begins to see themselves as a minority, not in a racial system, but in a power structure, then, they could grow collectively into a unifying force. According to Paulo Freire (1971), when a group of individuals acquires critical consciousness of being oppressed, and when they realize that they, as a group, are treated different or unfairly, they can become part of the world and act to change it.

Although the dominant discourse promotes and uses labels or identities based on assumed racial or ethnic differences, it does not mean that actual individuals take on those labels (Fraser 1989). Individuals such as these activists do have some freedom to negotiate how, if at all, and when to use the Latino identity. The ambiguity and contradictions characteristic of the

Latino (or Hispanic) label allow variation in the way people use it, and even the possibility of rejecting its use. Escaping a racial identity, however, is almost impossible in a society organized along racial differences.

The way individuals adapt to the dominant racial discourse in defining themselves is exemplified by nineteen-year-old Ignacio, who was born and raised in the Chicago area. As a child, he would help his parents read the bills, because they could not read English. Yet because his Spanish is limited, his high school peers would tell him that he was not a Latino. "I don't fit anywhere," Ignacio concludes:

> When I was in high school, I would always get, "Oh you're not Mexican."
> And I was like, what is it to be Mexican? People asked, "How come you never speak Spanish?" My own philosophy is, I'm Mexican and that has nothing to do with it. So in high school and in college, I distanced myself from the Latino community simply because I'd get shunned a lot, or I'd get a lot of "you're gay." But I feel very uncomfortable talking to Latino heterosexuals. I have this stereotype of Latino men, that I feel they're going to be very macho.
> Now, I'm in the moment of getting back into my Latino community. I know I could fit in. I want to see how I can better myself and how I can help that community, and work with the gay community too. I am Latino and gay, there's nothing wrong with that.

Both outsiders and insiders use Spanish language as a marker of ethnicity or race. After skin color, language is the most salient indicator of group membership. If someone is perceived as Latino, he is expected to speak Spanish. If he does not, he is not a "real" Latino. This may cause a conflict of identity for many individuals like Ignacio. He did not socialize with Latinos during his childhood and adolescent years. He felt rejected for two reasons. First, he did not speak the language. Second, he felt rejected because of his homosexuality. Now, as a young adult, Ignacio is working to become a "Latino" and incorporate the identity into his gay identity. Like many other first-generation immigrants from Latin America, he has sought out others to create and validate his own identity as a Latino. Yet, as Ignacio explains, this does not completely resolve the identity question, and he feels he continually has to explain to himself and others what Latino means:

> I think the term *Hispanic* is very Eurocentric. I think many people use that term not knowing what it means.
> So, I use *Latino* just to encompass everyone, "la raza de Latin America." I say Latino-Latina, and for me I'd say Chicano. That's my identity. I'm Chicano because I am American and I don't deny that. But I am Mexican too. I have to realize that, and I'm learning, but I don't fit in anywhere . . . I'm Mexican, but

I'm not Mexican. I will never be seen as a Mexican. Then I'm American, but I'm not white American.

Ignacio's struggle to make sense of himself in U.S. society and culture illustrates the interactive process by which individuals take on identities promoted by the dominant discourse. It reflects the dilemmas, conflicts, and consequences of adopting a label to define the self. Moreover, Ignacio's example shows the ambiguity and contradictions inherent in the label *Latino*.

In this chapter I present the way in which these activists live their lives as "Latinos" in a racial social system. In a parallel fashion to stigma related to gender nonconformity, I treat the racial labeling of groups as stigma. That is, to call someone Latino or to use the label *Latino* is part of the process of marking differences between groups, creating social separation, and establishing discriminatory practices. The stigmatization reinforces, if not creates, relations of power. From the viewpoint of the labeled group, stigma can take the form of actual experiences; perceptions about how others (or the society at large) see them; and internalization of the negative views others have in the self.

I begin with a discussion of the diverse forms of racism *compañeros* have faced. This section encompasses racism within the gay communities and in Latin American countries. I proceed with a discussion of the efforts of this group of activists to create a Latino ethnicity in the United States. Last, I present the process by which some of these activists have developed a critical consciousness as members of an oppressed minority.

The Experience of Race

One of the most lasting and painful marks of racism is, perhaps, the verbal and nonverbal actions individuals endure because they are considered different and inferior. Actions such as insults, segregation, and mistreatment leave permanent scars on the self. The size and severity of the scars may change as time passes, sometimes becoming invisible and numb. They never fade. They remain as constant reminders of who one is and of one's relation with the outside world. The scars define the way in which one sees oneself and the outside world.

The acts of racism also constitute the ways in which race is expressed and sustained. That is, when we insult a person because of her or his brown skin color, we are enacting race as the idea of difference. At the same time, we are reproducing the racial system that we live in and that gave origin to that insult.

Almost everybody in this group of activists has experienced racism at some point in their lives, whether they are immigrants or U.S. natives. Their experiences include insults, distancing or isolation, harassment, and mistreatment. Although these experiences are common, they are not as pervasive or salient as the experiences attributed to gender nonconformity. The latter are more numerous and painful to recount than the former. This is due to the relationship between the victim and the offender. In the case of gender nonconformity stigma, much of the stigmatization comes from family and friends. By contrast, stigmatization related to skin color or language typically comes from a distant other, such as teachers and classmates. Family and friends are rarely the sources of stigmatization.

Experiences of racism, like those of homophobia, are most common during childhood and adolescence. They are particularly salient as individuals enter the larger social world, that is, when children move from the usually monoethnic and monolingual environment of family and neighborhood to a multiethnic (if not majority white) milieu, such as school. Bilingual education is, unfortunately, a good example.

Abraham was born in New York City but spent some time in Puerto Rico. His parents were originally from the island. As a child he was enrolled in bilingual education because his English was not "very good." Like others who have gone through such a system, he describes this experience as "horrible":

> I remember having to be held back in a bilingual class. Bilingual then was horrible. It was in the basement and you were separated. You were just with a few other kids and it was like in the dingy room and it didn't make you feel really good.

The official discourse would say that the purpose of bilingual education, or any type of "special" education, is to promote advancement and integration. What Abraham experienced, however, is separation, which is a form of stigmatization similar to segregation. Separation can also be thought of as a social distancing between the "normal" students and the "special" or "not-normal" students. One consequence of this special treatment is the sense of being different from and less than others. As Abraham poignantly says, he was in a "basement." It makes children question their abilities and, furthermore, their sense of who they are. Because people like Abraham come to believe that others think they are not good enough, they strive to show otherwise:

> I always thought I had a speaking problem. I think those sorts of things created a lot of confusion. I used to think, "Am I smart?" I think it did affect me and I always had to prove that I was smart.

> Now my Spanish is horrible. It's almost like whatever I knew I forgot. This is the language that proved to be a major issue in my life, actually. It has a lot to do with identity.

Bilingual education not only separated Abraham from his peers and undermined his skills, it also made him question his Puerto Rican identity. The message Abraham received was that being Puerto Rican was not good. His problem was being Puerto Rican. Yet, in learning English, he lost his native language. Language is not simply a skill or a tool to communicate. It is the means by which culture is transmitted. It is the means by which a person constructs his or her world. According to Freire (1971), one comes to name and own one's world through language. This is why language such as "Puerto Rican Spanish" is the basis for Abraham's identity and the target of bilingual education in a racial system.

Although I have no data to generalize about the effects of bilingual education, the separation to which it gives rise has tinted the childhood memories of a few of these activists. Gabriel, for example, was brought to the United States when he was about a year old. When at the appropriate age he went to school in Salinas, California, he had to do first grade twice. Like Abraham, he "didn't know English" and had to take bilingual education:

> I remember how I used to get pulled out of my classes because I didn't speak English. I used to get individual help. I hated it because every day, at two or three, this Latino woman used to come into our classroom and say, "OK, we're here for the boys." It was always me, Jesus, José, Jorge. It was like all the white boys stayed—we had to go.

Gabriel's experience illustrates how bilingual education stigmatizes at the same time that it re-creates racial groups. First, bilingual education stigmatizes in that it separates individuals defined as "not-normal" (e.g., in need of help) from those considered "normal." Second, those labeled as not-normal are also not-white, while those defined as "normal" are also "white." This causes pain. Gabriel says, "I hated it." In this process, language, like one's ability to speak unaccented English, is closely tied to the idea of race, along with skin color. As noted before, language conveys individuals' identity and culture, hence its importance in the racial system for both the dominant and the oppressed groups. Still, this phenomenon is not widespread among *compañeros*.

Rejection is another form of stigmatization commonly experienced by these activists. This rejection is frequently the result of skin color and language, as demonstrated in the story of Abraham. Moreover, rejection usually comes along with insults, another form of stigmatization. The insult, or name-calling, is used to degrade, mark a difference, and, as a consequence, to reject. When a person is called a beaner, for instance, as Gonzalo illustrates next, he or she has been referred to as someone who eats beans and, therefore, is poor. Gonzalo says:

> I wasn't spoken to here because I was a Mexican. I was a beaner. That's what they would call me. So pretty soon, I learned to not associate with white people. When school was out, we moved to a city, which was bigger and more diverse.

Gonzalo was born in Mexico, where he spent his first years, in a very devoted Catholic family. His family came to the United States to improve their financial situation. When they arrived, they were the only family in town: the other migrant workers were all single adults. As a result, Gonzalo felt isolated at an early age. When he started school, he barely spoke any English, and none of the teachers were bilingual. "I felt pretty weird," Gonzalo recollects. "It felt isolated. I've never seen so many white people in my life."

Sergio also shared a story about an instance in college when he was referred to as a beaner. Sergio was born and raised in the United States. He is twenty-six years old and attended graduate school for a year:

> When I was in college, I was listening to Spanish music on my little portable radio. I had gotten up to go to the bathroom. When I came back into the room— my roommates were in the room when I had left—there were also two or three of their friends. I walked in. They didn't see me, they said, "Oh, there's the music, where's the beaner?" I said, "He's right behind you, you stupid son of a bitch."

The insults driven by language or skin color are very common. Only in a few instances, however, do these activists talk about responding to the insult as Sergio did. Confronting the offender can be difficult. It can be emotionally draining and may escalate into verbal and physical violence.

One last type of experience typically encountered by these activists is what may be called exoticism. It occurs when these individuals are made to feel or treated as exotic objects. A person is made exotic when he or she is attributed foreign, different, and frequently attractive (from the point of view of the designator or stigmatizer) features. These can relate to physical, personality, or character, and cultural traits. Again, Sergio provides an example of how this takes place in a college environment:

> I was the first one to move in[to] the dorm. The first roommate showed up. He was a really nice kid, with a really nice family from Massachusetts. That's why I called them the Kennedys. They were very liberal, but they also had sort of that white guilt. The liberal white guilt. The father was telling me, "Oh, what kind of name is Sergio?" And I said, "Oh, you know, it's Latin, my parents are from the Caribbean." "Oh, well, this will be a good multicultural experience for Matt." I'm like, "Oh great! I'm here to be someone's teacher."

Sergio was troubled by the comment because the roommate's father treated him as if he were different from his son. The father suggested that Sergio belonged to a different variety of people. From the father's perspective, he probably thought that he was making a compliment or being "liberal," stating that he was open to and accepting of different groups of people. For Sergio, however, the father's statement was indicative of his attitude that Sergio could be regarded as a strange object, which others can dissect and learn from. This exoticism is also seen in the context of sexual attraction and relationships between persons of "different races," or specifically, when a white person finds a nonwhite person sexually appealing. The next section deals with this issue.

The separation created by bilingual education, insults and mockery, rejection, and exoticism are part of all the adversity faced by these activists. These experiences are attributed largely to their skin color and language. They are some of the means by which the idea of race and difference is enacted. Being Latino, as Ariel puts it, "is in many ways like being gay. Is to be outside the larger society. Sometimes is harder than being gay. One can hide the gay part, but the color of your skin is very visible." In the previous chapter, we learned that Ariel tried to end his life due the agony he felt after realizing his homosexuality and leaving his church.

The experiences of stigmatization based on the idea of race, like those attributed to homosexuality, are particularly salient during childhood and adolescence. Stigmatization based on race is magnified when individuals leave the confines of a small and homogenous (e.g., same language and ethnicity) group, like the family and the neighborhood and enter a larger and mostly white setting. In the words of Ariel, "I didn't care about skin color when I was younger, maybe because I was in an enclosed and mostly Hispanic community. But as I step into the outside world, I notice it more. And I know that many people look first at the color of my skin."

These experiences of racism create isolation, distress, alienation (a sense of being different and not part of the world), and a sense of being less than others. The alienation and sense of inferiority reflect the internalization of the negative messages received from social institutions and the mainstream culture, such as schools and mass media. Such internalization sometimes is expressed by these activists as "having to prove" themselves to others. Once more, Ariel illustrates this clearly:

> My boyfriend tells me that I'm too hard on myself. "You're always trying to improve. Most of your friends are Anglo, and that's where I see it more." "Like you have to prove that you're an equal, or perhaps better than they. Like that's

what pushes you." I think he's right. But when I'm with a Hispanic group, I feel I can be myself without having to prove anything.

Having to prove oneself works as a motivation to do more and better than others because one thinks of oneself as less or undeserving. Sergio says: "Part of me still has the fire, desire, and will to strive and prove to people that I'm not here because someone handed me a check. I'm not here because affirmative action gave me a job or the chance to go to college." Having to prove oneself to others is one of most lasting outcomes of the U.S. racial system. It is still inscribed in Sergio's heart, despite (or perhaps because of) having a college degree and being a successful young professional.

Few of these activists have directly confronted their offenders. Although the majority of these activists do attribute insults or mistreatment to others' prejudice, few attribute such racism to their own flaws. They usually define the source of racism (or the racist comment) as an individual. In some instances, which are presented later in this chapter and in chapter 7, these activists identify social institutions or structural societal features as the sources of racial stigma.

The White Gay Ghetto

Humberto says that he never felt discriminated against because of his physical appearance until he moved to San Francisco and began visiting gay bars. "There's really, really a lot of racism," he notes. "It's not directed at you that much. But you feel it. Here, it's thrown at you." Now age forty-seven, Humberto was born in the United States and raised in California. In his teenage years, he was a victim of rumors about his sexual orientation in high school. As an adult, he speaks sharply about the rejection he has experienced in mainstream gay circles because of the perception that he is not Caucasian. His experience is not unique. Many of these activists speak of racial discrimination and segregation existing in bars, clubs, and organizations in the Bay Area, Chicago, New York, Miami, Washington, D.C., and other large cities around the country.

According to Humberto, the racist discrimination is not always overt. It frequently takes place in a more subtle manner. "You feel it," explains Humberto. It is perceived in the atmosphere created by the dominant presence of white men, the minimal interaction between white men and the few nonwhite men, and, in the words of Isidro, by the "body and gym culture."

One Peruvian activist, Felipe, suggests that the segregation in gay communities is not only based on skin color but also on social class:

> I'm not into going to the gay barrio. Everywhere, the neighborhoods are what
> I'd call white ghetto. A gay white ghetto. I'd even call it an upper-middle-class
> gay white ghetto. It is about race, but also is about social class. As a Latino and
> as a gay man, it doesn't do it for me.

Although other activists in this group would agree with this assessment, Felipe
is the only one who explicitly articulates it. This view is understood if we
recall that many of these activists are immigrants. Although some of them
hold middle-class positions, few of them can afford a lifestyle in the (mostly)
gay neighborhoods of Chicago and San Francisco. The cost of housing in
those gay neighborhoods is among the most expensive in the two cities.

Social class, thus, intensifies the segregation created by the idea of race in
gay communities. In the eyes and realities of *compañeros,* race and social
class converge to form a gay culture that is white and middle class. The
stigmatization emerging from such gay culture toward those with colored
skin and broken English has isolated and alienated many of these activists.
Yet, others participate in the dominant gay culture and, in some instances,
employ the widespread racialized views of Latinos to their own advantage.
One example is the use of their "Latino" characteristics to attract white gay
men. They take advantage of the exoticism. Luigi describes:

> When I lived in San Diego, I started meeting white men who liked my eyes, my
> hair, and my cock. They liked the way I looked; my hairy body. I played that
> for a while. I don't play it any more. I want to be seen as an entire person now.

Luigi's approach to play the "race card," so to speak, is somewhat contradictory. On the one hand, it reproduces the stigmatizing attitudes toward
Latinos. To a large extent, it normalizes the use of the "race card" as a
part of the gay culture and its stigmatization toward Latinos. On the other
hand, Luigi is conscious about the fact that he is playing the "race card."
He knows that he can use it when he so desires. He also is aware that such
an approach is objectifying and racist. Thus, he has some control over the
act of being objectified. Because of that, the stigmatization may not be as
damaging at the personal level as an insult could be.

Color and Class in Latin America

In Latin America, color and social class generally concur. People with light
skin color are found in the upper social strata, while those with dark skin
color such as blacks, mulattoes, or mestizos are found usually in the lower
social strata. There are exceptions, of course. Social class, however, seems
to have more power than skin color to define one's position in society.

Growing up poor in Mexico on the outskirts of Mexico City, George also had the misfortune of being "moreno"—that is, a dark-skinned person. When he finished elementary school, his father decided to send him to a good junior high school because of George's good grades. Since the junior high school was on the other side of the city, George had to travel an hour each way by bus and metro to get there. Going to this new school was, in George's words, a "trauma." It was not traumatic academically but socially and psychologically. Most of the youths in this school came from middle-class families. George was poor and from a "lower social class." "I'd see them in their shining shoes and nice cleaned and ironed clothes," says George. In addition, most of these youths were "güeritos" (fair-skinned and blond hair). George was the target of insults, which made him become withdrawn and isolated.

George's experience in his new school is indicative of a common pattern, by which light-skinned individuals are a part of the middle and upper social classes in many Latin American countries. George says, "There is discrimination regarding social class, but when you're *moreno* or shorty, the kids reject you too." George also notes that he did not feel different when he attended a school in his neighborhood, which was a small poor settlement just outside the city. When he began venturing into the larger world, he was made different. He became poor and *moreno*. George realized that others had better clothes and shoes and lighter skin than he did. Then, he experienced isolation.

Another activist, Ramiro, was the "negrito de la familia" (the black kid in the family) in Brazil. His family used to call him "negrito," a term of endearment. In the United States, he could easily be referred to as an African American or black. Growing up in Brazil, he never felt that his skin color mattered, because his family was financially well-off. As a child he did not have any black friends, and he attended a private Catholic school where "everybody was white." In the school, "I never felt any different," he notes. "I had money, and people knew who I was." Thus, skin color in many Latin American settings is relevant, but it may be nullified by social class. Ramiro further explains:

In Brazil, I was dark-skinned, but I had a father who had money, so it was never an issue. And being the darker one in my family, there was always that tender joke, the *negrito*.

Finding Latinoness

The racial social structure leads many of these activists, especially those born and raised in the United States, to seek out other Latinos and search and re-create their origin or past. That is, they work to create their ethnicity by means of learning Spanish, joining Latino organizations, having Latino friends, and learning about their family's past and country of origin. This is the result of the alienation in the Freirian and Marxist sense brought about by racism. As members of a dominated group, the language, history, and culture in which they lived and are educated are not of their own making. This creates what Octavio Paz (1962) called *soledad* (solitude). For many of these activists, their adult lives and their activism are efforts to fight that solitude.

The solitude is expressed by Pablo when he says, "Growing up, I was always with Caucasian people. I grew up kind of whitewashed. I wasn't really exposed to the real Mexican way." His activism through several organizations in San Francisco has led him to meet other Latinos and even a boyfriend who is an immigrant from Mexico. Joining an organization that provides services and support groups for Latinos has helped Pablo "feel at home" and "feel like I belong there." In other organizations with which he was involved before, he frequently felt as the "only Latin in the room":

> I'm realizing who I really am. Now, because I'm involved in these different areas, I've got to learn I'm Mexican. It's helped me immensely to open up to my own culture. I always kind of felt like an outsider, even though I'm Mexican, I still feel like an outsider looking in, in a Mexican room. But now I feel like I'm part of it.

In Pablo's story we see a trajectory from growing up "whitewashed" as a consequence of time spent around white people to learning to be a Mexican in his adult years. Retrospectively, he describes the early years of being in someone else's world—or, the world of Caucasian people. He grew up in solitude. What is also significant in this latter phase of Pablo's story is the idea of learning a culture and identity: "I got to learn I'm Mexican." This idea is frequently expressed among other activists born and raised here. It is also articulated among other groups such as African Americans, when they try to recover their ancestry on the African continent prior to slavery in America. To learn a culture and ethnicity one thinks one belongs to, or an identity that one thinks is of the self sounds "unnatural." To learn who one is seems unnatural when seen from the viewpoint of those activists who are immigrant and were born and raised in Latin American countries. Their culture, ethnicity, and identity (e.g., based on national origin) are taken for granted and perhaps never even talked about, except when they migrate to other countries, such as the United States. For them, culture and identity are lived rather than actively pursued and learned. Thus, the notion of learning to be somebody or a culture is possible in U.S. society, which is structured around the idea of race.

Some immigrants also talk about facing alienation, since they do not fit neatly into the established racial or ethnic groupings. For example, Ramiro, the activist from Brazil, has become acquainted with a group of Latinos through his activism. Despite the language differences (Ramiro's first language is Brazilian Portuguese), he has been able to identify with the mostly Spanish-speaking Latinos:

> It was very hard for me to connect with African Americans and with white men. Having this organization is like half of the home. Even though the language is not the same, I think the religious and sexuality aspects of life are very similar. Our dynamics, our happiness and sadness are very similar, more so than African Americans' and white gay men's.

Although Ramiro's skin is black, he could not identify with African American groups. And although he is gay, he could not associate with white gay men. Ramiro could relate, however, to Latinos born here and with immigrants like himself from Latin America. With them, he was able to share and express his religious beliefs and sexuality in a comfortable manner, just as if they were "Brazilian men." It is in instances such as this one that ethnicity and a sense of shared culture are created and maintained. In the face of solitude, many of these activists claim a shared culture, constructing themselves as an ethnic group.

Yet learning about ethnicity, one's identity and the celebration of them is frequently tinted with romanticism. Aspects of one's culture such as country of origin, holidays, music, and customs are commemorated with some nostalgia created by the distance of time and space. What some of these activists practice as their identity or ethnicity (e.g., Mexican, Puerto Rican) is in fact an abstraction of the original or a reinterpretation of the actual culture of their country of origin. This romanticism is observable for some of these activists when either visiting their parents' country of origin or when they encounter an incompatible feature, such as stigma. Gerardo, an activist from Chicago, was disappointed when he visited Puerto Rico, his parents' homeland, for the first time. After troubling initial years in school, he was "reconnecting" with his Latino heritage in high school. In this process, he visited the island:

> I had never been in a school with so many Latinos. I was just like "Man. *¿Qué pasó?*" [What happened?] I really reconnected with being Latino and with being different.
>
> It wasn't just that I was an American, I was a Puerto Rican American, and I wanted to know this place that my folks came from. My dad would take us there. He was like, "When school's over, you're going to go to Puerto Rico to live on that farm with your grandparents." "Great. No running water! We're out in the middle of nowhere and you want me to ride a horse. I want a man on a horse to come and get me and take me away from all of this."

Growing up in Chicago, Gerardo had all the amenities that even some working-class families have. He did not find those amenities in his parents' and grandparents' farm and small town in Puerto Rico. Still, he claims, and with pride, a Puerto Rican identity. He wants to remember, however, not to relive his ancestors' origin. The place of origin is a poor and isolated place, without the comfort that even many racial minorities in the United States enjoy.

Abraham also experienced disillusion when he visited Puerto Rico. In his youth he began studying "Latino history" when he realized the alienation that he felt because his formal schooling never exposed him to Latino culture and history. While studying art, he would read books on Latin American and Puerto Rican history. He says, "I was really interested in my own history." Then in the early 1990s, he became involved with a Puerto Rican cultural organization in Chicago. "I was already investigating the whole thing about my identity and being Puerto Rican." Abraham began to travel to Puerto Rico. Now, he feels "more Puerto Rican than in Puerto Rico." On his latest trip, he realized there was a significant amount of "Americanism." "There's people that listen to rock and rap. It wasn't always that strong in the youth culture; now, it is." To some extent, Abraham has to overcome his alienation. He feels Puerto Rican and has visited the island several times. His identity and image of Puerto Rico do not mirror what he experiences on the island.

Making connections with other Latinos is difficult for those who do not speak Spanish. Language may constitute a difficult barrier to overcoming the solitude created by being labeled differently. Jack, who is living with HIV, has had such an experience in his efforts to relate to other Latinos. He grew up in the Midwest, with English as his first language. His only contact with some aspect of a Mexican culture was in his childhood, via his grandparents. "It was good to go there on Sundays and have *barbacoa*, rice, beans, and to listen to Mexican music." Now in his midthirties, he has embraced his Latino identity:

> I don't remember ever feeling like I really belonged to any one community, even the Latino community. I feel like I'm outside, because of my language.

The Creation of Consciousness

Paulo Freire (1971) defines critical consciousness as the ability to see the contradictions of the social world and to act to change them. It implies seeing the self as a part of an oppressed group and a product of social circumstances. Some *compañeros* have this type of perspective. They do not necessarily see themselves as a racial or an ethnic group, but as a part of a disadvantaged or oppressed group. One activist, Rigoberto, who is perhaps one of the most involved from Chicago, actually uses Latino as an overarching concept, regardless of national origin or race:

> I think *Latino* is more of an umbrella term. It identifies me with a whole group of people, just like *queer* does. I don't identify myself as American. I mean I don't usually use that term. This is a country where slavery was openly practiced, where people were lynched and hanged; treaties with the Native Americans were violated, and treaties with Mexico were violated.

Rigoberto, whose father is an immigrant from Mexico, uses the Latino label and identity with a political agenda. In his use, the term implies power relationships between groups of people. The American represents the powerful, whereas the Latino, like himself, is the oppressed. Some of these activists trace their understandings of race and Latino to their upbringing and experiences in college. Noel, for example, attributes his understanding of racism to his experiences as a child in Central America. Noel is a forty-five-year-old, HIV-positive activist in Chicago:

> I come from a country in revolution, where people were fighting for human rights. So, since I was a child, I knew that discrimination was wrong. There was always talk about our origins and about indigenous people. And I know that the problems with identity come from issues about race, because some people are taught that having indigenous or black blood in you is not good. My family taught us that we were *mestizos*. When I moved here, I noticed a lot of discrimination against Latinos. To start, I have the title of Latino for the first time. Back in Latin America, I did not have it. But when you are sure about your identity, you see why things are not working well and then you can do something about it.

Sergio thought of himself as a "minority" for the first time when he was in college. He is twenty-five years old and grew up in Florida in a neighborhood of immigrant families from Latin American and the Caribbean. It was not until college that he felt "very different." He attended a private, mostly white college outside of Florida. There, he underwent a transformation:

> When I graduated from high school, I was much more shy, quiet and just not really sure of myself. By the time I finished college, I was obnoxiously sure of myself. College gave me a new sense of identity. I grew up in a Latin family. I was surrounded in my neighborhood by people who looked like me, who talked like me, and who ate the food that I ate. Then I get to college, a predominantly white school. I was one of two graduating Latino males. So it gave me a militant side about myself, and sort of an anger that there are people in this world who have things that others don't.

The anger was not about "I'm going to go punch a wall," but the type of "I'm going to protest; let's go take over the student union; let's go institute a black studies program, because it's been 20 years since they were trying to do it."

Before his college experience, Sergio did not know what minority meant. He did not see himself as minority. What triggered his critical view and activism was a peer mentor that he met through a special program at his college. The mentor was a black woman. She and her boyfriend were active in campus politics. Sergio calls them "the most militant people I probably will meet in my life." Sergio got involved in campus organizations and protests through them. He learned "that you can ask for something and if you don't get it, you have to do a little bit more than ask; you have to show them that you're not asking, you're demanding." On his college journey, Sergio developed an understanding of Latinos as a minority. Minority was not about numbers, but about access to resources. Sergio's view of minority, thus, echoes the Marxist's view of social class.

Like Sergio, Armando went through a transformation in college. He grew up in California and went to college in the Northeast. Unlike Sergio, Armando tells a story of growing up internalizing racial and homosexual stigma. As a child and teenager, he was troubled by being poor, Latino, and gay. To avoid having to confront those identities and the stigma associated with them, Armando joined a gothic group while in high school:

> I was in middle school when I was concerned about being poor, and being perceived as poor by the kids. I remember internalizing my gayness. Also internalizing my Mexicanness and Latinoness. During high school, a certain part of me didn't want to be Mexican, didn't want to be gay, and didn't want to be Latino. I wanted to be this kind of dark, artistic, gothic industrial kid.
>
> But, in a way, it was just like a facade to keep me away from dealing with being Latino, and being perceived as a loser or gang member, all the things that are negative about Latinos and about fags.

During those years, Armando even had little contact with other Latinos or Mexican immigrants. He was perceived by them as "white-washed" or a "sell-out." In college, however, he began what he calls his "awakening." He credits this to his involvement in gay, Latino, and African American groups. His education on "radical theory" was likewise a contributing factor:

> I became aware of the struggle of both populations, gay and Latinos, and came to embrace it. I was pretty involved, politically, in college with the Latino club groups and in protests about the college threatening to close down the Latino and African American houses. I was pretty involved with the gay groups.
>
> That, in conjunction with my education, helped. I took a lot of democratic,

radical theory, and radical queer theory. I read a lot of Marx's socialist theory. About how a lot of your life depends on your social and economic status. That was a big awakening for me. I understood where I came from, why I was afraid of being Latino.

While in college and far away from his home and family, Armando was able to bring together the Latino and gay aspects of his life. The stigma that he had internalized as a child now was attributed to the social environment. He began feeling comfortable with those two spheres, enabling him to participate in campus groups and protests. Moreover, he developed a critical consciousness. Like Sergio, Armando infused his understanding of Latino with Marxist theory. He saw himself not as an ethnic or racial minority but as a member of a disadvantaged group. His position in society was defined, at least in part, by access to resources.

Renato, a thirty-eight-year-old activist, sees Latinos as an oppressed group. Closely echoing Freire's ideas, he sees oppression as the factor linking not only race, or racism, but also homophobia, stigma toward HIV-positive people, and Puerto Rico's dependence on the United States:

> I strongly believe oppression is oppression. I think a lot of the issues that we deal with in HIV education or antihomophobia work are behind racism. Maybe I'm a little taller or light skinned. I don't experience the oppression that others do. So, if you're black, there is no way that anyone would not think you are black. I think the issues that are behind that type of racism and the oppression experienced by black or by Latino people, are exactly the same things that are behind homophobia, or behind HIV.

Recently, Renato, who is living with HIV, also became involved in Puerto Rican politics through his church group. He participates in a small group in San Francisco supporting the liberation of political prisoners on the island. Before this, he was not aware of the Puerto Rican independence movement. He explains that he, like many residents in Puerto Rico, did not know what the "United States's colonialism and imperialism has done to Puerto Rico."

To have a critical consciousness about oneself as a member of a group named Latinos means, for this small group of activists, to be part of an oppressed group. This oppression is based on access to resources, such as education, income, and housing. Oppression, for some, could also be based on skin color, or the idea of race. This limited access to resources goes beyond skin color, permeating sexual orientation and HIV/AIDS status.

This critical consciousness about being Latino is part of the activism of *compañeros*. It is difficult to ascertain whether that consciousness is a cause or an effect of their activism. For some, their consciousness led to activism; for others, activism created a critical consciousness; and for others activism further developed an incipient consciousness. In their stories, however, we noted some elements that contribute to the development of such consciousness. These include family upbringing or education; college experiences; peers and mentors; and participation in students' organizations as well as community-based organizations working for either ethnic or gay-related issues.

The elements contributing to the creation and growth of a critical consciousness work, to some extent, by nullifying the internalized stigma. Many of these activists have been exposed to racial stigmatization (along with that based on gender nonconformity). Some of them internalized such stigma, incorporating society's negative views of Latinos into their self-concepts. They turned the stigma from the inside to the outside partly through their exposure to the above noted elements, such as college education and activism. Now the stigma is attributed to the social, not to the self. The stigma toward Latinos is nothing more than societies' own misconceptions and one of the means by which oppression is sustained. The response to the insults, discrimination, and other manifestations of stigma is not silence or self-pride, but social action to change the immediate social environment.

CHAPTER FOUR

The Formation of Gay
and Trans Identities

To become a gay or a transgender person is, still, an act of rebellion. The rebellion is against the power that asks us to follow the predefined gender roles of a man or a woman. The force that compels us to think, act, and desire as a man (in the case of those biologically defined as males) or a woman (in the case of those biologically defined as females). That force comes through family, school, religion, media, law, and state policies.

The act of rebellion, however, does not lead to freedom, or the newly found freedom is not boundless. As one rejects the assigned gender role, or the expectations of parents and religious doctrines, and takes on the identity of "gay man" or "transgender," one is agreeing, to a degree, to another set of expectations and norms. One is complying with a set of rules about how and what to think, act, and desire (Foucault 1976/1990; Scott 1986; Sawicki 1991; de Lauretis 1987; Ewick and Selby 1995).

In this chapter I describe how *compañeros* came to call themselves gay or transgender (from male to female). As with the Latino label, not all the activists refer to themselves as gay or transgender. Some call themselves queer, while others refer to themselves as either drag queens, women, or simply use female pronouns when talking about themselves, especially in Spanish. Moreover, these categories deployed to define the self are socially constructed. Actually, to name same-sex desire between men "gay" is a relatively new phenomenon (Chauncey 1994). This identity, which stands as a third identity next to woman and man, is the product of social and political forces in the early and mid-twentieth century in Western Europe and United States. The gay man identity, thus, emerged as the primary way to name same-sex desire and as a way of living for a group of white males in affluent societies. Toward the end of the twentieth century, the gay identity became widely spread in countries like Mexico and Brazil (Carrillo 2002; Parker 1991).

The life histories of these activists show that the adoption and construction of a gay and transgender identity is largely a sociocultural process in which peers, community organizations, and other socializing venues, such as bars and neighborhoods, play a central function. These activists adopt identities as gay or bisexual men and transgender as they meet *compañeros*: peers who share their experiences, mentor them, and support them to overcome the internalized stigma. In the words of Pierre, a Cuban immigrant living in Chicago, *compañeros* help see one self "inside out" and "knock down the wall" of repression.

Becoming a Gay Man

"I Was Born Gay"

When asked about how they became gay or when they first thought of themselves as gay, these Latino men say that they were born gay. They, of course, did not mean that they have always called themselves gay or that they always knew they were gay. What they do mean is that since an early age they felt different from others. They saw themselves as different from other boys, and they knew they related differently to other males from how they saw other boys relating to males. Also, they saw that their parents and schoolteachers treated them differently from other male siblings or friends. As Victor, the twenty-three-year-old activist from Chicago, explains, "I've always known it. When I was a kid, it was like I was ridiculed, so I'd push it away." Some of these men articulate this feeling of being different as not fitting traditional gender roles, such as not liking to play soccer and wanting to play with dolls. Others, however, did not express the sense of being different in those terms. They simply intuited that something about them was distinctive.

Fabian "came out of the closet" ("salir del closet," he says) at the age of thirty when he decided to divorce his wife. He has always felt different, however:

> I always was very different. . . . I think it was that I've always been gay. Although back then I didn't know what gay meant, I knew I liked men, since I was little. I believe I was five or six years old. Of course, I didn't know how to verbalize it. But I knew it wasn't correct that I was attracted to a man; I felt guilt.

At the age they start feeling different from other boys, these men cannot name or articulate their emotions. But they can learn moral values. They begin to distinguish good from bad. Hence, as they begin to experience distinctive emotions from those expected by their assigned gender, they start attaching negative meanings to those feelings. They learn to hide such emotions to avoid negative reactions from others, as we have seen in the stigmatization of gender nonconformity.

The expression "I was born gay," used by many *compañeros,* is also a response to the discourse that defines same-sex desire as pathological. Medicine and psychiatry (despite having removed the label of disease from homosexuality in the United States and the Americas), in particular, have helped popularize the idea that there is something inherently wrong with homosexual or transgender persons. Accordingly, they suggest that some-where along the way in a gay person's development, something went wrong, be it an unresolved Oedipus complex or sexual abuse that "caused" same-sex desire. This is the discourse that prompts the "why" question: Why are you homosexual?:

> I knew [I was gay] since I began walking. Many people think that I learned it or that I was raped. But it is something I cannot change. It cannot be changed. I cannot be someone I'm not.

Jimmy felt "different" since he was a little boy in Mexico. "Different in the sense of being gay," he clarifies. As he tells the story of how he came to see himself as a gay man, he seems to address the larger society and medicine and psychiatry's discourse. Jimmy emphatically notes that he was not social-ized into homosexuality or sexually abused. Those are not the causes of his homosexuality. In fact, implicitly he says that there are no causes.

In the stories of becoming gay, "being born gay" marks the beginning of a journey in search of the self. Being born gay does not mean one knows who one is, wants, and desires since childhood. It means that one feels dif-ferent from other boys. That difference, however, cannot always be defined or named. This difference sometimes takes the form of crossing gender boundaries in games, toys, clothing, and behaviors, or attraction or fondness toward other males. In such cases, the difference is further demarcated by stigmatization, when others prohibit or discipline those behaviors or desires. The stigmatization, in turn, leads to repressing that sense of being different.

Later in life, sexual encounters and "messing around" with other men bring about contradictory feelings. On the one hand, they produce excite-ment and satisfaction. On the other hand, they increase confusion, create remorse, and are concealed in secrecy. Alberto, for example, says that his first sexual encounter with a man left him "scared" and thinking he was doing something wrong. At the age of sixteen, Alberto met at a city park a man a couple of years older than he was. They went to the man's apartment, where they had sex. "Of course, I was very nervous. But I was very excited about it too. The thought of doing it excited me." Alberto had been "playing around" with other males of his same age since he was eight years old. But this was his first sexual intercourse. After sex, the man asked Alberto to meet again. Initially, Alberto was enthusiastic about the idea of having sex again, but later the guilt he felt made him change his mind. "I left thinking, 'Oh God, what am I doing? I can't do that, it's wrong.'"

Yet the guilt and remorse escalate as the frequency and intensity of sexual encounters with other men increase and as these men move from adolescence to adulthood. "I felt inferior," Marc recounts his feelings about having sex with a man. "I felt dirty and low. I felt like everybody was looking at me, as if they knew what I had done. In my mind, I was being chased." The guilt and the attraction to members of the same sex give rise to crisis and to a subsequent struggle.

An intense struggle created by the conflict between the outside world and the self ensues. These men understood (and many still do), rightfully, that the outside world stigmatizes same-sex desires. Many of them had internalized such stigma. That is, while a part of them wanted to enjoy their same-sex desire, another part condemned such desire. During this struggle, they endure deep emotional feelings, such as depression, loneliness, and suicidal behavior. The outcome of this struggle, in most instances, is the realization and self-acceptance of their homosexuality. This outcome, however, is not immediate.

Entering Gay Life

The struggle between the self and the outside world does not completely end when these men accept their homosexuality, call themselves gay, or tell others that they are gay. It does not have a clear end point, and for some the struggle continues throughout their lives. But as these men begin to find ways to confront the conflict, the process of self-acceptance begins. This process of self-acceptance, in most cases, refers to the adoption of an identity as a gay man. The turning point is the change in the attribution of stigma from inside to the outside world. The negative perception begins to be shifted from the self to the prejudice of the other—family, church, and the larger society. Two connected elements activate this process: self-reflection and contact with gay culture through peers, organizations, and bars. Other gay men, LGBT organizations, and bars provide the social support and framework for *compañeros* to begin to see the gay-man identity in positive terms.

Like many teenagers, when Marc was about twelve years old, he was spending more time with his friends and at school than with his family. When he turned sixteen, however, Marc began to feel rejected by his friends because he did not act as most young males do in Peru, his homeland. That rejection led him to seek out other friends:

> As I grew up, my friends started suspecting about me. They started having girlfriends and I didn't having any. "Why don't you have a girlfriend?" I began to separate from them because I felt pressured by them.
>
> It became clear I was homosexual and some of them distanced themselves. So I did the same, drifted apart, because I said, "What do I do if they only want to talk about girlfriends, talk to them about guys?" So I went out to bars and other places, outside the barrio, to find guys from the *ambiente,* gay guys.

In meeting other gay men in the bars and parks of Lima, Marc realized he was not alone: "I'm not the only one—there are others like me." The exposure to other gay men provided the social support for Marc to feel comfortable with his homosexuality and, as he explains, "not to get lost":

> I felt comfortable knowing I was not the only one. Then I began to accept myself a little more. The beauty of that moment is that everything becomes open, all is revealed, you can do things with other men like you want.
>
> I met gay people, *del ambiente,* I knew where to find them. I'd have gotten lost without them. So knowing other people helped me understand who I am, know myself, and accept myself little by little.

Among the new friendships that Marc created was with an older man, a college professor, who guided Marc through the process of accepting himself as a gay man and overcoming the shame and guilt Marc felt every time he had sex:

> I'd feel like it was the worst thing I had done. [After sex] I never felt happy. This friend, who was a bit older than me, told me that it was normal, that I shouldn't feel guilty for doing what I like to do, that I had to accept myself.
>
> I began to accept that I'm gay and that I like men. . . . I knew who I was and I knew I had to work on accepting myself and fighting my religious values. I had to accept myself, the way I was, as a human being, as I was born. So I tried to meet gay friends and see that I wasn't the only one.

The vast majority of the activists living in San Francisco were born and raised elsewhere. Some of them came to the city in search of themselves. Others, somewhat unintentionally, found their gay identity in the city after witnessing the normalcy and richness of the gay communities. Seeing other gay men going about their everyday lives helped some of these activists realize that, in the words of Hugo, "there is nothing wrong." Hugo is thirty-two years old and the son of a Native American woman:

> I've been in San Francisco since 1985. I was a teenager when I came here with my family. I've been here ever since. It was a big difference from where we came from, Arizona. When I came here, I came out as a gay male. I saw gay people living normal lives and I came to terms with my sexuality. I saw that there was nothing wrong with being gay.
>
> Before coming here I had sex with a couple of people. I was about thirteen. It made me unsure of myself because I figured morally that it was wrong. I didn't know what was wrong with me. I still knew deep inside that I was gay, but I just didn't come to terms with it until I came here and I saw the gay community.

Many of the *compañeros* who immigrated later in their lives to San Francisco came to avoid the stigmatization that their families, and society in general, attached to homosexuality in their homeland. They did not see a viable future for themselves in their home country as gay men. Employment, for instance, could become tenuous if they shared their identity publicly as they grew older. Cohabitating with another man could likewise lead to further stigmatization.

Other *compañeros* came to accept themselves as gay thanks to gay peers they met in their workplaces. Ismael and Alberto tell stories of finding gay men with whom they felt comfortable enough to express their homosexuality and subsequently enter into the gay culture. For Ismael, acceptance of his homosexuality and introduction into gay social circles also coincided with his first sexual experience. Ismael was born and raised in Mexico but migrated to Chicago in his early teenage years. He was nineteen years old when he met Steve, who was twenty-six:

> Steve and I started hanging out a lot at work. Then he took me to a friend's party. It was a gay party. I had never been late at home, so that night I told my mom I was going to be a bit late. I got to the party and felt very comfortable, like never before. I was able to be like I wanted to be.

That was the first night that Ismael did not sleep at his parents' home. Because he was drunk, Steve took him to his place. The next morning, Ismael called his mother to apologize and explain to her that he got drunk the night before and stayed at a friend's home.

Alberto, a forty-seven-year-old activist from California, was just out of high school and working at a fast-food restaurant when he met Dwayne. This, Alberto says, was "the turning point. I came out of my closet, and this guy brought me out." Dwayne and Alberto were working together and felt a mutual attraction. They began dating, but what was most significant for Alberto is that Dwayne took him to a gay bar for the first time. Alberto was eighteen years old:

> We dated just very briefly, but he is the one that pretty much brought me out, took me to my first gay bar. I had never really known any other gay person. So when I walked in this place and I see all these other guys like me, just kind of average, and they weren't queens. My impression of gays at that time was always that they were all queens and drag queens.
>
> This is during the early '70s, when the gay life was still pretty underground. I walked in and saw all these guys. It was like, "Wow, this is great!"

Like Alberto, many of these activists talk about not wanting to look like "queens." They want to relate to men who look "masculine," which for many is the "normal male." As shown in Alberto's story, this is particularly relevant in youth, when these men are in the process of constructing their sexual identity. The stigmatizing image that they have internalized tells them that being effeminate is erroneous. Part of the struggle for acceptance comes from the stigma society attaches to a man who looks like a woman. Thus, when they see gay men who do not act feminine, they think of them as acceptable and as models for their own homosexuality. This look is less likely to create negative reactions from others than the feminine; hence, they tend to adapt such a look for themselves. They want to be "normal," and to do that they have to reject the image of a man dressed in woman's clothes. They distance themselves from the "queens" and transgenders.

Orlando, a Chicago native living with HIV, met other gay men in college when he was thirty years old. He had been in psychotherapy a few times, but meeting peers made "a world of difference" for him:

> I met other people who felt good about being gay. I think it makes a world of a difference when you run across people that went through very similar things; like, OK, it's normal. It's fine [to be gay] and maybe that's the way I'm supposed to be.
>
> I remember this group of guys up at the university I hung out with. Their mission was to turn me out. They took me to a gay bar. I had a blast! I remember, "Oh, this can't be bad. I'm not hurting anyone." I think a lot of it was just important social support among new friends from school.

As for Fabian and Mario, who married women, their entrance into the gay culture, and, hence, their adoption of a gay identity, was not very different from that of the men who remained single. There are only two differences. First, they came to terms with their homosexuality later in their lives than most men. Second, as a consequence, their struggle was extended for several years and it implicated other people, including their wives and children, in addition to their parents and siblings. The experience that they share with others is that what triggered their adoption of a gay identity was their contact with gay culture and LGBT organizations.

Fabian was still living in Mexico when he got married. After years in therapy, he dated his wife-to-be for six years. The first couple of years, they had sex "every once in a while." Although Fabian enjoyed it, the frequency declined as years passed. During those six years, Fabian had a few sexual encounters with men he found cruising. "I didn't want to accept that I was gay," Fabian says of the reason he got married. He did not want to lose his girlfriend and thought his attraction for men was temporary. They got married and moved to the United States. The marriage lasted two years. It prolonged Fabian's struggle and brought unhappiness to both Fabian and his wife. The marriage was plagued with difficulties due to Fabian's repressed homosexuality and the stress of their migration to the United States:

> Our marriage wasn't good at all. We weren't happy. We rarely had sex. I began to realize that I really liked men, so I felt bitter, depressed. I didn't know how to find a way out of it because I loved her and I didn't want to hurt her. I didn't want to hurt my family.

It took Fabian three months to find a job in Chicago, while his wife did clerical work there. They had little money and their new apartment was bare, except for the bedroom. One weekend, as they were exploring the city, Fabian found the mostly gay neighborhood:

> We were walking through the city, a Saturday afternoon, and we noticed that there were a lot of men in that area. Obviously they looked gay. We saw the bars too. So I knew where the gay area was, and I started going there and meeting men.

It is still painful for Fabian to recall this period of his life. He feels responsible for the failure of his marriage and guilty for the lies and his wife's pain. While his wife was at work, Fabian frequented the gay neighborhood and eventually became involved in a sexual relationship with another man. Fabian says they only met a half-dozen times for sex, but meeting this person made Fabian see gay life as a possibility:

> It helped me to meet this guy, because I met someone who was living openly as a gay man. I started to realize that it wasn't wrong to be gay, that there are many gay people doing OK with their lives. That this doesn't mean to live alone, it doesn't mean people would hate you. All the prejudice began to go down little by little.

Fabian was altering the stigma that he had internalized. The reality that he witnessed in Chicago did not match the negative stereotypes associated with being gay. This set off the process that would cause Fabian to divorce his wife and take on an identity as a gay man. After the affair, Fabian found a job and there he met another gay man. This time, Fabian fell in love. The relationship grew stronger for several months, until Fabian's coworker ended it because he did not want to continue hiding the relationship. Determined to change his life, Fabian contacted Horizons, the largest LGBT organization in Chicago (now named Center on Halsted). He attended several therapy sessions and then talked to his wife about his homosexuality. Fabian divorced his wife. Five years later, they remain close friends.

For his part, Mario was married for eighteen years. During the course of the marriage, he had two children and moved with his family to the United States. Mario's main reason for getting married to a woman was his family's deep involvement in a Protestant church. He wanted to follow "las buenas costumbres"—an allusion to Carlos Fuentes's now-classic novel *Las buenas conciencias (The Good Consciences)*. He left the marriage when he found out that his wife was having an affair and was in love with his close friend. He arrived in San Francisco, where he contacted Aguilas (eagles), a Latino gay group:

> I have gone through a lot of stuff, but I can't live hating myself. I lived looking for a key. A key to find out what it was that I was feeling and wanting. "How come I can't get an erection with a woman?"
>
> I found it through this group. It's because of the six years in this group that I can now speak of myself as I do.

Mario discovered his identity as a gay man in Aguilas. He learned the language to accept his homosexuality through the group, which also enabled him to make sense of his life. Now fifty, Mario lives in San Francisco and sees his teenage children frequently.

Entering gay life for almost all of these men is marked by relief and joy. When they meet empathetic friends, are able to express their inner feelings and desire for other men, and begin to find a place for themselves, they feel supported and free.

Coming Out to Family

After entering gay life and meeting peers, adopting a gay identity in the midst of family, especially parents, is the most difficult process for *compañeros*. Many of these activists, indeed, have opted not to take on a gay identity with their families of origin. Coming out is part of the process of creating an identity. As gay men explain to others their sexuality, they create a language to make sense of the self. This language for explanation is also acquired through peers or organizations.

Telling parents about one's homosexuality frequently occurs only after one has told friends. It is more difficult to tell parents than friends, because the consequences are potentially more severe with the former. These can include rejection and cutting off all ties with the family. That is part of the reason many of these activists have not talked directly about their homosexuality with their families. Among those who had, the circumstances of their coming-out vary and the reactions from family members also vary.

Julian's conversation with his family happened impromptu. He was born and raised in Mexico. In his youth, he emigrated to San Francisco after moving to Chicago from Mexico with his parents. Living so far from his parents, it was easier for Julian to live openly as a gay man. He and his partner lived together for a few years without his parents' knowledge. When they visited Julian's parents, he was caught in the middle: his boyfriend did not know Julian's parents did not know about him, and Julian's parents, of course, were not aware of their son's life in San Francisco.

> My dad was very serious. "Who is he?" "This is Jim, the guy I live with in San Francisco." Still my father was checking him out all the time. And we stayed with them. Night came and my father goes, "This is the room for you and that is the room for you." Jim then said, "We can sleep together, not a big deal, we do it all the time." My dad got serious but only said, "Whatever you want to do."
> I was hoping Jim would go to the other room, but he stayed with me.

The next morning, Julian's mother asked why they sleep together in San Francisco. Julian told her that the apartment was very small, and they could not fit two beds. Then, Julian told his parents, "I want to talk to you guys." He sent Jim to take a walk while they talked:

> I told them I wanted to be sincere, but that I needed their understanding. My mom asked, "What's going on?" I said, "I have lived a gay life since I was sixteen. In Mexico I was more reserved, but here in the United States I felt more freedom."
> My dad said to my mom, "I told you I didn't want him to come here [the United States] because it'd be a mess."

Julian's father did not take the news well and did not talk to Julian for a year. His mother, on the contrary, did not mind, and expressed her support to him. "I love you as you are and nothing will change that. Take care of yourself. I'm always with you."

Like Julian, many *compañeros* lived dual lives for many years, and some still do. They keep their lives as gay men separate or a secret from their families of origin, especially if they live in different cities or countries, mainly because of the stigma toward homosexuality. One of the reasons they disclose their homosexuality to their families is to bring together their divergent lives. They get tired of making up stories and hiding. They also want to be able to share their lives with their families. Some accomplish it, others only partially, while still others fail in their attempts to unite their gay identity and their roles as sons and brothers.

Unlike Julian, Ignacio, who is only nineteen years old, was angrily confronted and slapped by his mother:

> They were in their bedroom, watching TV. "Mom, Pa, I'm gay." They're like, "What?" So then the TV goes off and the lights go [on]. My dad is very passive. My mom is mad, "Qué estás diciendo?" [What are you saying?] I said, "Yes."
>
> I never cried about being gay until that moment. My mom was the one who said, "We didn't raise you like that." She says, "Quieres que te meta un palo para que te haga gay?" [Do you want me to shove a stick in you to make you gay?].
>
> "How could you do this to the family?" She told me I needed to see a psychologist or a counselor. Then I got pissed off. "You know what? I am fine. There's nothing wrong with me. If there's something wrong it is with you. You're very ignorant about homosexuality." She goes, "Yeah, you're going to die of AIDS."

Two years later, Ignacio's parents participate in Ignacio's life and accept his homosexuality. This is largely due to Ignacio's efforts to involve them and inform them about gay events and activities. Ignacio talks to them about his friends, his activism, and other gay events, like the Pride Parade. His mother even attended a ceremony in which Ignacio was awarded a fellowship for his activism with Latino gay men. "We got dressed up and stuff and I took her. She was happy and she laughed."

Creating a gay identity within the family may also involve an educational process. The education is aimed at developing a positive image, for both the son and the family. As many families do stigmatize nonconforming gender behaviors, including their sons', some of these men take the initiative of changing their families' stereotypes. Eric, a forty-six-year-old Puerto Rican activist living in Chicago, explains:

> We are twelve in the family; everybody's different; I have to use different approach methods. Some of them accepted it, others cried and wanted me to see a psychiatrist. I explained to them that being gay wasn't bad. I let them know about my success in life and all my achievements.
>
> I educated them about gay issues, about what being gay is and that not everybody is bad or going to bed with everyone.

The educational work these men engage in is aimed at achieving acceptance within the family, at being seen and treated as any other member of the family. The stereotypes are replaced by the image of a son, who is brought into the

family rather than thought of as a distant other (e.g., the homosexual). Many
of these men who have revealed their sexual orientation have succeeded not
only in being accepted by their families but also in changing their families'
negative attitudes toward gay men. Fabian's story illustrates this point:

> I sat them down in the living room and told them that I was gay. I told them
> I had separated from my wife. It was hard for my parents, more for my dad
> than for my mom. He was depressed for several days.
>
> But I [had] thought about it, [and] I had planned to stay the whole week
> with them, so I could talk to them, educate them, and help them. They are very
> liberal and opened-minded, but the culture in Mexico is so homophobic that
> you soak it up.

Fabian later got them some books on gay issues that he ordered from Spain.
They were the only books he could find in Spanish. Over time, both of Fabian's parents changed, and two years later, Fabian visited his parents and
brought his partner. The most visible change, however, was in his father:

> My dad told me: "I never thought that this late in my life an event would trans-
> form me so much, that it'd make me grow so much." He says he has grown and
> has realized that he has discriminated against others.

According to men whose families are aware of their gay identities, involvement in gay communities and access to gay-related resources helps them
face their families. After being estranged from his family for a year, Eduardo,
an activist living in San Francisco, "came out" with his family a few years
ago. At thirty-four years of age, Eduardo was active in gay organizations in
San Francisco. But his family, living elsewhere in California, did not know
about his life in San Francisco. He explains that the separation eventually
began to hurt him, so he decided to talk to his family:

> I thought, "All this pain that I'm in is coming from my not being out to my
> family." Here I was living in San Francisco and going to gay bars, having gay
> sex, volunteering in gay organizations, working in a gay office—my mom had
> no idea about any of that aspect of my life.
>
> I thought that all the problems I was having were stemming from me not
> being out. I wanted to see if coming out to the family would change things.

Eduardo felt motivated to break the silence with his family because he
was missing their support and was feeling incomplete. He then consulted
a therapist and several books, including Rafael Díaz's book on Latinos
and HIV (1998). These resources helped him approach his family:

> I went to see a therapist and I told her about my family, that I wanted to come
> out to them. I bought a book on coming out, which didn't really help much.

Then I read the book by Rafael Díaz. It was really helpful. I just really identified with a lot of what he was saying.

In a similar predicament with his family, Isidro found the courage to talk to his mother from ACT UP and the Coming-Out Day celebration. He had moved out of his mother's house in the Bay Area in his late teens, after his mother questioned him about his sexual orientation. At that time, Isidro told her it was "just a phase." That was his way of dealing with his mother's question and his new life living with a male friend. Isidro developed gay friends in the Bay Area and got involved with ACT UP. A year later, he called his mother on Coming-Out Day to tell her he was gay:

"You know, I am gay, blah, blah, blah." And she said, "OK, well, I feel better knowing that my kids can come to me with anything and not have to worry about anything, but don't tell your dad."

Despite these stories, we must not conclude that a person has to construct an identity as a "gay man" in public and in the family to develop as an individual and function in society. In the same way we do not equate same-sex desire with a gay identity, we should not assume that a gay identity has to be laid over all spheres of an individual's life, or that sharing such identity with the family always has a positive result. We live in a time and place (the United States in particular) in which sex and sexual behavior are thought of as the source of one's identity, and in which individuals are encouraged to "confess" or make public their identities. Hence, the popularity of the "coming-out" ritual or disclosure of one's sexual orientation among lay, professional, and academic communities. The ritual has become so ingrained in the gay culture that it has reached the level of a moral issue so that those who are not "out" and are "in the closet" are criticized and thought of as dishonest. This is evident in the way in which some of these activists speak about sharing their sexual identity with their families. Vladimir, for example, speaks of "confessing" to his Mexican siblings and parents that he is homosexual and of "being sincere" and "not deceiving" them about his life.

The stories of becoming a gay man represent a search for the self. They trace how these men have been searching for an identity that can provide the channel to express themselves. Collectively, these stories tell us that the pursuit begins early in life, with an unnamed self. As children, these men felt different from their peers and unable to fit the assigned gender roles. Their thoughts and actions crossed gender boundaries, but they did not think of themselves as belonging to the opposite gender. They thought of themselves as within their assigned biological sex and gender role. Their social milieu did not provide models for them to identify. They were given only the traditional gender models of man and woman, with their associated expectations. It was not until their youth and early adulthood, when they met peers and groups, that they found the language to make sense of their difference and tell their own stories.

In their stories, most men adopt the contemporary identity of gay man. With rare exceptions, some identify themselves as homosexuals, bisexuals, or queers. Although some men criticize the gay culture as being "white," that is, not representing the experiences of ethnic minority groups, most men do feel comfortable calling themselves gay. This reflects at least two social processes. One is the dominance of the gay identity, not only in the United States, but in many Latin American countries. As Hector Carrillo (2002) notes, the gay identity as created in the United States and Western Europe has expanded to communities in Mexico and coexists with other, and perhaps older, identities and labels, such as those based on the gender system. None of these men speak of themselves in terms of "man," "woman," "feminine," "passive," or "active," which reflect a gender-based system to label the self. Homosexual men, thus, are defining themselves more on the basis of their sexual attraction than in terms of the traditional gender roles.

The second process is the part these men play in LGBT and AIDS activism. To a large extent, their identities as gay men reflect the membership and agenda of those organizations, as it will be seen in chapters 6 and 7. The stories about becoming gay are the product of their own reflections and the stories they have encountered among their *compañeros*.

"The Woman That I Am"

To become a woman when one was given a male identity and socialized as a man is an act of defiance. It entails breaking the cultural law that states that genitalia equal gender. Transgenders (and transsexuals as well) show us that our gender roles are not defined by sex. They illustrate that gender is not defined by an immutable essence (Mason-Shrock 1996). Their presence suggests that we might just be able to be whomever we want to become. I say "might" because, paradoxically, the transformation from male to female is not made in a free-will space and, hence, must be accompanied by a cautionary note. Transgender persons frequently rely on taken-for-granted ideas about gender (e.g., what is to be a woman and a man) to construct their stories and to create their newfound selves as women.

While different from accounts of becoming a gay man, transgenders' narratives of transformation share some features with the former. Transgenders, like gay men, speak about feeling different from early childhood and being stigmatized for not conforming to their assigned gender. They also speak about sexual games with other boys and sexual experiences in their teen-age years. What is different from the gay experience is the cross-dressing in childhood, the intensified stigmatization, the absence of the coming-out ritual, and the emphasis on the process of transforming the self from male to female. And, of course, the outcome of the transformation, an identity as transgender, is different from that found among gay men.

Cross-dressing and Sexual Games

Contrary to the stereotype, not all transgenders in my study tell stories of cross-dressing early in their lives. Almost all of them note, like gay men do, that they felt different than other males from the time they were little boys. But only about half of the transgenders cross-dressed when they were boys. Angelica, whom we met in chapter 1, is one of them. Angelica recounts that she "was always very feminine." As a child, she would try on her sisters' clothes. "I've always liked wearing girls' clothes. When I was little, I used to try on my sisters' clothes all the time." For Angelica, cross-dressing then was a game. She did not do it again until she was in high school. Then, she realized she wanted to live as a woman full-time.

Blanca grew up in California in the 1940s, a couple of generations before Angelica. When she was a child, she would try on women's clothes with the help of an aunt. "The kids made fun of me and called me *joto,* but I still wore the dress." She would also put on lipstick and makeup. Blanca would pretend she was performing in a theater, singing and dancing conga, like Tongolele, a famed Mexican female dancer; María Victoria, a famous Mexican singer and actor; and, of course, Lola Beltrán. Blanca would eventually become well-known in the Bay Area for her performances as a female ranchero singer. As a little boy, she notes, "I was already a screaming faggot. 'I want to come out, the woman that I am!'"

Sex, in the form of games or actual intercourse, is another recurring element in the transgenders' childhood accounts. Thalia's first sexual experience, at the age of ten, is not rare. Many *compañeras* had sex for the first time sometime between the ages of five and twelve:

> It was with a *muchachito del barrio* [neighborhood boy]. We went out, sup-posedly to play soccer in the park. And that's where everything happened. He was thirteen and I was ten. We had sex. I liked it; he knew I was gay. He had more experience, so he told me, "Come this way."
>
> I went and there he told me, "Let's fuck." "But how?" I asked. "You'll see; I'll show you how." That was the first time I had a *relación* [sexual intercourse].

Thalia had sex with that teenager a couple of times. Later, she would have sex with a male cousin.

The Transformation

The teenage years of this group of *compañeras* are marked by an awareness of their sexual and romantic attraction toward other men and the beginning of their male-to-female transformation. Sex is no longer a game or something that just happens to them. Sex is desire, romance, and, sometimes, dishonor:

> As I grew up, I realized I was gay. I had no one to tell I was in love with this or that guy. I always liked them older and with a big moustache. I dreamed they were making love to me. With time, I knew I was homosexual and that people didn't take that well; that being gay was horrible.
>
> I felt in love two or three times. This particular guy was handsome, *simpático* [pleasant], and nice. I felt taken care of. He introduced me to his family. But that was platonic love; I never had sex with him. Because in my youth and adolescence, I was conscious that I was gay, so I was embarrassed to tell him anything, like, "I like you." I thought they'd go away or tell others in school, "He's gay, *un puñal* [faggot]."

The stories of the teenage years also hint at the adoption of gender role as women. We find traces of the prevailing social meanings of woman, such as playing the receptive role, rather than insertive, in sexual intercourse and being emotive (e.g., falling in love). These features are not as predominant among gay men and provide continuity to the creation of a role as a woman, which for some transgenders began with cross-dressing in childhood.

These activists actually use the term *transformation* to describe the process leading to living full-time as a woman. In a manner similar to that of gay men entering the gay life, peers and role models trigger this transformation process.

Carmen began her transformation when she found a "teacher" in Mexico City. "The transformation was very difficult," she notes. She grew up in a small town and in her teens she moved to Mexico City. There, she visited a bar in La Alameda park. It was a bar "de ambiente," frequented by homosexual men. "I was in my 20s, and I started hanging out with them. Some of them really wiggled their hips, and I was embarrassed—'how dare you do that!'" Later, Carmen shared her apartment with a friend she made at that bar. Carmen began to emulate her friend. "She'd pluck an eyebrow, I'd do too; she'd wear a shirt with a flower, I'd have one with five flowers. That's how it went, until I decided to dress up as a woman." Carmen felt comfortable dressing as a woman, but she was harassed by the police: "they see you; they catch you and send you to jail."

Carmen also met a "maestra" (teacher), a male-to-female transsexual who taught her how to dance and do female impersonations. "She showed me how to dance rock and roll and *cumbia*." Carmen enjoyed performing, "singing like Lola Beltrán," either for free at friends' homes or for pay in bars. Then she let her hair grow long, depilated her body, and slowly changed her work clothes from blazer and tie to blouse and high heels.

Carmen's transformation story is similar to the stories of gay men, in that the construction of a new identity emerges from the interaction with others who either already have created an identity (e.g., woman, transvestite, transsexual) or are in the process of creating such an identity. Through her peers and teacher, Carmen learned how to dress, act, and perform as a woman. Through them, she also developed the confidence to change her outlook in public and defy stigmatization. Carmen is now fifty-one years old and lives in San Francisco. She is not taking hormones and has not had any surgical procedures to change her gender identity.

The basic elements of the transformation process were the same for Angelica, who at twenty-five is half Carmen's age:

> It was my junior year, I went to school in drag for Halloween, but it wasn't like totally femmed out. And then I didn't dress up for about a year. Then I started meeting more queens and just getting more into the scene. I started going out dressed up. And I liked that.
>
> For a while I struggled with my daytime, 'cause it's very important to me to work. I had started taking hormones and stuff. But I was still living as a female only at night. Then, during the day people would start calling me Miss. I was like, "Wow, OK, these meds are working." 'Cause I wouldn't wear heavy foundation. I just wear powder in the daytime. I've been very androgynous. So, I was like, "I need to start working as a female."
>
> I decided this past year, actually, on International Women's Day [annually on 8 March], was the first day that I went to work. I'll put on some makeup and do it. I wanted to do it for like six months to a year before I started taking hormone therapy. So right now I'm not on hormones. I just dress. For me it's also like resocialization. It's psychological and emotional too.

When Angelica began dressing as a woman during the day, she was living in San Francisco. She explains that she had taken some hormones a few years ago but stopped taking them to undergo a medically supervised hormone therapy. A unique aspect in Angelica's life is the acceptance and support she has received from her family. Her family knows about her transformation and has witnessed it for the most part. Her siblings, but not her parents, call her by her female name.

Thalia also lives in San Francisco. Two years ago, she started her hormone therapy under the supervision of a psychologist and a physician. Her transformation, however, had a troubled beginning. After leaving her home and family in Mexico City, she worked in the sex industry in the United States–Mexico border on her way to San Francisco. At the border, she found work in a cantina. There, the other transgenders (more precisely, transvestites) working there and the woman supervising them dressed her and put on her makeup. She liked the way she looked. When Thalia moved to San Francisco as a teen, she contacted her high school counselor to talk about her desire to dress as a woman:

> I felt supported in the school. The counselor told me that I wasn't the only one or the first one in the school or the city. He told me this is a gay city and that the law protected me. So I started little by little, putting on a little bit of makeup, letting my hair grow long, then more makeup, until I dressed as a woman.

Some male students would make fun of Thalia at school. But then she found a small group of gay, queer, and transgender students, who were brought together by a teacher. "We made everybody in the school respect us. Nowadays nobody says anything, whether you go as a woman, male, or gay." Thalia's body and voice are changing now. "My voice is higher now and my face is finer." Her goal is "to become a complete woman," and she plans to continue hormone therapy and undergo surgery.

Among this group of transgenders, the significant generation gap makes their stories a little different. Carmen and Blanca grew up in the 1940s and 1950s, while Thalia and Angelica grew up in the early 1980s. Carmen and Blanca speak about "performing" as a woman, female impersonation shows of famous Latin American singers, and police harassment. They refer to their peers in female terms but don't label them as transgender or transsexual. They speak little of hormone therapy, psychological support, or surgery. In contrast, Thalia and Angelica talk about hormone therapy, psychological counseling, and transgender peers. Although the essence of the transformation is the same across all their stories, those subtle differences reflect important historical changes in the construction of identities. The identities presented in the stories of Blanca and Carmen are of males performing as females, or men playing the women's roles. That is, their identities are not transgender, in the strict sense of the term. In contrast, the stories of Thalia and Angelica present an identity of a woman, not of a male performing as a female.

Compañeros and *compañeras* are a fundamental element in the stories about becoming a gay man and a transgender person. They come in the form of friendships, role models, or boyfriends. They are found in a public park, a café, a gay bar, a community organization, or at school and they trigger the formation of identities. *Compañeros* provide company, a common history, and a shared oppression. They supply a language to name the previously unnamed desire and sense of difference.

The identity, thus, is created in the company of others. Here is where identity intersects with volunteerism and activism, particularly in HIV/AIDS and LGBT organizations. We can not establish a causal order between joining and creating an identity. We can not say what came first, joining a community organization, or calling oneself gay or transgender. A few of these men and transgender persons joined an organization as volunteers or activists. In doing so, they constructed their identities as gay men or transgender. That is, they joined and then found themselves, in large part due to the peers and resources in the organization. Several others became activists or volunteers only after they defined themselves as gay men or transgender. Yet many of them joined organizations and groups to find peers who could support a sense of self, provide a community, and fight together against oppression. Chapters 6 and 7 explain the process of joining in detail.

CHAPTER FIVE

LIFE WITH HIV AND AIDS

HIV triggers a transformation of the self that may lead to activism. The transformation, however, is frequently painful and slow, and activism is not its immediate outcome. Fear, shame, illness, and depression usually come before. This change and the stories that we are about to read come about in large part because of the advances in the medical treatments. Even as recently as 1990, these stories would not have been feasible. The medical treatments, commonly known as HAART (highly active antiretroviral therapy), along with the services of AIDS organizations, have prolonged the life expectancy and improved the quality of life of those living with HIV and AIDS so that we can learn about their stories.

In this chapter I focus on the experiences of those *compañeros* who live with HIV or AIDS. I make the distinction because, although all of the activists in this group have HIV, less than a half of them have been diagnosed with AIDS. These activists have a vested interest in the progression of the AIDS movement. HIV and AIDS pushed them into activism to fight for their lives. All of them initially got involved in the AIDS movement because of their own encounter with HIV and AIDS.

Andres, who is fifty-three years old and has been HIV positive since 1985, says that AIDS is to gay men what the Holocaust is for Jewish people. "We have so many martyrs. Many had to sacrifice their lives for others to survive." For many gay men, Andres explains, AIDS has meant not only illness but also a loss of personal talents and friendships. HIV and AIDS have been yet another force to contend with. Gay men and transgender persons are locked in a struggle to live and be themselves.

But they refuse to see themselves as victims. Paradoxically, they seem to have so much life running through their veins—the same veins through which the constant threats of suffering and dying run. As seen in this chapter, they continue to fight, while the frequent visits to doctors, regular blood tests, and daily medications remind them of their mortality and the shame they must face in having a condition for which some people have no compassion but only condemnation.

Fallo Positivo

"Fallo positivo" denotes getting a positive HIV test result. "EL Fallo Positivo" is also the title of a famous song by the Spanish group Mecano (1991). This was the first song to introduce the idea of HIV as a personal tragedy into the young Spanish-speaking popular culture.

Gregorio grew up in southern Mexico and is thirty-six years old. In the following excerpt, he echoes a conclusion shared by many researchers and public health professionals across the United States: Latino and African American gay men come to know they have HIV, and sometimes AIDS, only when their health is already weakened (CDC 2006; Brooks et al. 2003; Needle et al. 2003; MacKellar et al. 2005). They learn they have been infected by HIV only after the virus has caused significant damage to their immune system. This is the case among most of these activists. Most of them got the devastating news after falling ill.

> In '96, I turned HIV positive. It was in a situation that even these days is very common. It's typical among minorities not to be tested regularly. People get infected and live without knowing it for many years. So it gets to the point that when we realize it, it's under already difficult conditions.

Gregorio learned he had AIDS only after entering the emergency room at a public hospital:

> It was wintertime and I came down with a cold. A cold that wouldn't go away. It got so bad that I eventually started having breathing problems. I asked my roommate to take me to the hospital.
>
> This marked a change in my life. I recall they told him, "We'll give him medical attention." I recall being put on a stretcher and taken to a surgery room. I recall seeing a light. I was like dead, I lost consciousness. I woke up three or four days later. I had all sorts of equipment around my body. I had a tube going through my nose that even left a mark in my nose. I saw two of my best friends standing beside me, I cried. At the same time, it was comforting to see them.
>
> It was a difficult situation. The doctor had called my family and told them my condition was severe and that I could die. I didn't know he had talked with them. Then, I recall being taken to the recovery room.
>
> Then, a medical student told me, "You have a type of pneumonia that is

common among people with HIV. You know you're HIV positive, right?" I told him "no."

That was the moment Gregorio learned he had HIV. The news overwhelmed him to the point that he considered taking his own life. But he found strength in his relationship with his mother, even though she wasn't there with him physically, and in the support of his friends:

> The impact was such that I thought about suicide; to throw myself out of the window. But I think what kept me and gave me strength was my mother. Even in the worst of times, I have been close to my mother.

The support of family and friends (which I explore in detail later in this chapter), are critical elements for activists in their fight against HIV and AIDS. With the help of a friend, Gregorio had gone to the hospital, where the presence of two of his close friends gave him an "internal peace" and the image of his mother restored his desire to live.

Gregorio left the hospital with a verbal AIDS diagnosis as yet unconfirmed by an HIV test. He returned two weeks later for the results of his HIV test. "I had a sense it was positive," he recollects. Gregorio had brought a friend with him and asked the counselor if his friend could be present during the meeting. "He is one of my best friends. I want him to be with me." Gregorio's tests results confirmed the diagnosis: he had HIV and AIDS. By then, however, he was not thinking about killing himself. "What I need is education. I need to learn about this. I need to know where I can get some assistance."

With just two weeks elapsed since learning he probably had HIV/AIDS and since contemplating suicide, Gregorio was ready to fight back. With the support of his family and friends and the help of a medical regimen, Gregorio started looking for resources to fight AIDS so that he could return to the life he once had. Gregorio's story is testament to his resiliency—his ability to bounce back and be proactive.

Ramón was not concerned about HIV before he was told he had AIDS. He was divorced from a woman with whom he had two children, and he was living with his children and his mother. As in the case of Gregorio, Ramón disregarded HIV and AIDS messages that he would hear in the media, largely as a defense mechanism. He felt invincible: "It won't happen to me. I'm Superman." "But then," he recollects, "I got candidiasis." Candidiasis is an infection that frequently causes white patches in the mouth:

> I thought it'd go away in a few days. But it didn't. I got scared. I went to see the doctor. I saw her face changing. "You got AIDS," she told me. My world fell apart. "How much life I got?" That was the first thing that came to my mind.

Ramón had to compose himself and appear as if nothing had happened for his mother and his children. "I entered with a smile on my face. 'I'm home, Mom.'" His children were already in bed. Ramón went to his bedroom to be by himself and cry. Jokingly, he says, "Mary Magdalene's tears fell short," in allusion to the popular religious image of Mary Magdalene's weeping at Jesus' tomb. Ramón spent all night crying and thinking about his future: "What am I going to do?" "When am I going to die?" "My children are so little."

As the sun was rising, Ramón had an idea to call the AIDS hotline. He called the operator in search of the phone number. When he got it, he hesitated making the call: "They would know who I am. They would know everything about me:"

> God bless the woman who answered the phone. She asked me, "Did you get the HIV test?" "No," I replied. "No need to worry that much yet. . . . If you take care of yourself, you'll have a long life." She gave me all the information I needed.

A couple of weeks later, Ramón learned his HIV test was positive. The moment of clarity he had, when he thought about calling the hotline, was a turning point. He did not wait for depression and pessimistic thoughts to take over his life. He acted quickly and with determination. As will be seen later in this chapter, Ramón joined a support group for people living with HIV and founded another group with the help of other Latino men.

Among this group of activists, Jack is the only one who did not feel ill before knowing he was HIV positive. In the late 1980s, when Jack was twenty-one years old and living in the Midwest, he was tested for HIV. He was told to come back for a confirmation test. Jack did not go back. "It scared me so much":

> I remember at that point dropping to my knees and saying, "God, if you're out there, use my life, show me what this means, I don't want to go back." I remember crying. So I just went into denial and just said, "Screw it."

Three years later, Jack took another test because the possibility of being HIV positive still nagged at him. When the doctor told him that his T-cell level (part of the immune system) was very low (around 225), Jack realized that the first HIV test he took must have been positive:

> At that time, we still were dealing with the fear of dying. I wanted to live my life to the fullest. I wanted to do God's will. I wanted to make an impact in life.

Jack had an inner desire to live, fight HIV, and get involved in his community, as the other activists did. This has been part of his life to this point, more than a decade after learning he was HIV positive and that his immune system was weakening. Part of that inner desire to live stems from his spiritual orientation. Jack turned to his faith for strength when he was confronted by HIV.

The story of Mateo is different. The vast majority of the activists living with HIV and AIDS entered community activism after learning they were HIV positive or after suffering with AIDS. By contrast, Mateo was already involved in the AIDS movement and, before that, in the Roman Catholic youth movement. He had been participating in HIV/AIDS prevention groups and organizations in Mexico, where he grew up and lived until he immigrated to Canada and then to the United States in search of medical treatments.

The news about being HIV positive was not particularly devastating to Mateo. "I think it helped me a lot the fact that I was volunteering with groups supporting people living with HIV and AIDS." Mateo was in relative good health, kept himself informed, and had seen how others were dealing with HIV and AIDS. This helped Mateo to face HIV with a positive attitude:

> There is a solution for everything. We are mortals. So, in the meantime, enjoy your life, while being cautious and having safe sex. But there is no use to getting depressed and frustrated.

Learning that they had HIV, and for some also AIDS, was demoralizing for most of these activists. Many of them received the diagnosis when they were already experiencing some illness, but being ill was not as distressing as the fact that HIV caused the illness. The virus was a death sentence in the late 1980s and early 1990s and even more recently in the minds of many of these men and transgender persons. Moreover, HIV and AIDS carry stigmatization as not many other health conditions do; they are seen to be related to homosexual sex, anal sex, drug use, and "irresponsible" behavior.

The Support of Family, Boyfriends, and *Compañeros*

While learning about these activists' battles with HIV and AIDS, we have glimpsed the support provided by family members, friends, community-based organizations, and their social-support groups. These, along with religion and spirituality, coalesce in the resiliency of these activists. Family, friends, community-based organizations and support groups play a unique and important role in these activists' efforts to cope with HIV and AIDS.

In order to tap into the support of these sources, people must disclose their HIV or AIDS status. To find support necessitates offering the reason why such support is needed. Disclosing one's HIV or AIDS status is, as expected, difficult because of the stigma attached to it. The illness may bring shame and rejection similar to the stigma related to gender nonconformity.

Jimmy became ill in New York City, where he was living by himself. His sister and brother came from Chicago to take care of him. When Jimmy eventually moved in with his sister in Chicago, the siblings informed their mother, who lives in Mexico, and flew her in. Jimmy's brother and sister were crucial in his recovery. In Chicago, they dealt with hospitals and doctors, took care of him, and gave him a home. Jimmy's mother, however, gave him the strength to fight AIDS:

> She came to see me and it really helped me. It gave me the strength to move on. I told myself, "I can't give up. I have to show not to the world, but to myself that I can do it."

The doctors informed Jimmy's relatives about his condition and HIV/AIDS diagnosis when he was unconscious and ill in the hospital, so he was relieved of the burden of that disclosure. Jimmy has never encountered any type of rejection from his family. He says:

> I thank God that my family knows what I have. . . . It is sad that we had to go through such a painful experience to see us as a family. They supported me and still do.

Mothers have had a constant presence in these histories. Earlier, the figure of the mother was present as a caregiver, guardian, and accomplice. Now, mothers often provide the support and strength *compañeros* need to fight HIV and AIDS. Jacobo, who lives in San Francisco, talks about his mother's support:

> My mother accepts me and she loves me. She knows I'm HIV positive and supports me, even though she is getting very old, she comes from a rural area and had very little education. Right now, she is a very important part of my life.
>
> She encourages me, "Son, we all are going to die. When? We don't know. So, trust in God and ask him to guide you and to help you go on."

Jacobo even brought his mother to his social support group in San Francisco. She attended the group to talk about her relationship with her son and about how she has accepted his sexual orientation and dealt with her son's HIV status.

Another activist, Carmen, decided to disclose her HIV status to her mother after hearing a testimony similar to that offered by Jacobo and his mother. Carmen says that she was in a group when another member, a Latino man, said, "My mother knows, and from the moment I told her, she has become my best friend." That comment resonated with Carmen. She asked a friend to join her, and both flew to Mexico City, where Carmen's mother lives. Carmen explains that she needed the support of a friend to find the courage to speak with her mother. Her mother did not reject Carmen, though she asked her not to tell her extended family: "they might see you with disgust," her mother cautioned.

Peers and support groups likewise occupy a prominent place in the lives of these activists. Jimmy, for instance found support in a local AIDS organization that works mostly with Latinos. During one of his hospital stays in Chicago, he met a man who told him about the services provided by the organization. Jimmy was interested in going but afraid of walking in by himself, so he asked the man if he could take him. Jimmy went and since then has participated in a social support group:

> I met many people; lots of people who have been living with this for many years. I told myself, "Wow, and here I'm feeling like dying." Some of them have lived with this for up to fifteen years. I realized that I wasn't alone. I also realized that I was wasting my time with those depressions.
>
> The *compañeros* helped me. "I have lived so many years and also thought about dying. . . . It's normal what you're feeling." They encourage me and give me hope.

In this support group Jimmy found a community. He found people who were in the same situation, or who have had the same experience. That is, he found *compañeros*. The group provided him with a frame of reference through which to evaluate himself. In the process, it gave him hope. He learned that others have lived many more years with HIV and AIDS than he has—hence, probably enduring more pain than he as well. Furthermore, the group helped Jimmy normalize his illness. Through the shared experiences, Jimmy was able to understand his depression, mood changes, aches, and struggle with medication as a part of his illness and as normal events among those living with HIV and AIDS.

Compañeros are recurring characters in the lives of these activists. They too played a defining role in the identity development of these activists. They helped them in becoming gay men and transgender persons. Now, they reappear and perform similar roles. They care, validate, and encourage. They provide information, share experiences, and build self-esteem.

While searching for services for people living with HIV and AIDS, Gregorio found someone he referred to as a *compañera*. She did not have HIV but worked for a social services organization and took him to a support group. Gregorio felt connected to the group from the outset:

I found in them a desire to live and to do something for the community. Many of them were volunteers in the organization and very outspoken. They became my role models. They spoke about their condition openly, with no shame.

Support groups thereby provide a space for expression. Being among peers helps express oneself by enabling the acquisition of the vocabulary and the confidence to name one's condition and share it with others. Moreover, Gregorio and many of these activists have found their role models and *compañeros* in support groups. They show them how to deal with HIV and AIDS as an actual health condition and how to fight it in the social sphere as activists.

Boyfriends and partners are also a source of support in facing HIV and AIDS. Although less prominent in the support role than mothers, family, and peers, they are often the persons with whom these activists are most intimate—hence, they are the most immediate resource. For example, the Peruvian Marc says that his boyfriend gave him the "strength to go on":

> When I became positive, I thought I'd die in two weeks. I'd go out and see people on the streets but they had no value for me anymore. I'd be crying all the time, thinking I was about to die.
>
> He [my boyfriend] helped me a lot; I had nothing. I had no job and he told me, "Don't worry, you'll have what you need while we figure out what to do with this illness." I felt very supported—without it, it would have been devastating for me.

At that time, Marc's boyfriend did not have HIV. Marc does not think that he got HIV from his boyfriend. Incidentally, Marc has not told his family about his health condition. He has revealed his status only to a small group of trusted friends.

Marc then found a support group for Latinos with HIV through the AIDS Foundation of San Francisco. As evidenced with previous cases, Marc found a community when he felt abandoned:

> I felt like I was the only person who was [HIV] positive. When I went to the group, I found a lot of friends. Some of them were actually friends of mine, who had never told me they were positive too. We'd be very careful about our privacy.

Marc therein highlights another quality of the support group: it is a safe place. Unlike our relationships with friends, acquaintances, and coworkers, support groups usually have an explicit confidentiality rule. What happens in the group and the identity of the participants stays in the group. This ensures that people who are vulnerable to stigma for whatever reason can reveal their conditions and express themselves freely. This is part of what makes a support group a safe space.

The assistance and the comfort offered by peers and boyfriends have also helped some of these activists to disclose their status to their families, and, in turn, gather their support. For some *compañeros*, disclosing that they have HIV or AIDS to their family members can be very difficult. They fear rejection and shame. Their fears are sometimes intensified because their families do not know about their sexual orientation, or they have not explicitly discussed their sexual orientation with their families. Disclosure is frequently a more stressful decision and event for those who live with, or are close to, their families than for those whose families are either in another city or another country. The concealment of HIV and AIDS puts stress on family relationships and may eventually undermine them. It may also affect the health of those living with HIV or AIDS, because they have to hide medications, laboratory tests, and doctors' appointments.

When Ramón tested positive in Chicago, the counselor referred him to an AIDS organization, where a social support group for people living with HIV and AIDS was about to be formed. The following week, Ramón went to the group. He was hesitant, though. He recalls standing in front of the building, where he stood asking himself, "Should I . . . ? Should I go in? What would they say about me? What if they want to know stuff about my life?" He walked in and, as others have discovered, met a small community where he could express himself openly and be understood:

> I went in. I didn't want to leave! I met a lot of beautiful people. I felt I could talk about everything without being singled out or criticized. I did not want to tell my family.
>
> [In the group] I shared a lot of my experiences; I saw that I was not the only one; there were a lot of us. I felt better. I talked frankly.

After several months, Ramón felt he was ready to talk with his family. He lived with his mother and his two children, so he could not keep his secret for long. It had become a heavy burden for him. "I had to tell somebody because I didn't want that weight on my shoulders and I wanted to tell someone in the family." Ramón chose to talk to his older sister first. Her reaction was positive. She was not aware of Ramón's homosexuality, however. Ramón seized the opportunity to tell her that he was gay. "How could that be if you have children?" That was his sister's initial reaction. "You're my brother and I can't reject you. I can't. You have been with me in the good and the bad times. Now it is my turn."

Ramón's sister also encouraged him to speak to the rest of the family. Her argument was that they were a family, a unit, in which each member needed the other. "This is a family and what happens to one the rest have to know it. This is something that not only affects you. It affects all the family." With the help of his sister, then, Ramón informed all his siblings and his mother.

Ramón chose to talk to his two teenage children individually. He first talked with his daughter. "She cried like Mary Magdalene. But she told me she loved me and she supported me." It was a little more difficult for his son than for his daughter:

> My son took it differently. He was serious and didn't say a word. I felt very bad, like the whole world had collapsed.
> I cried and, then, fell asleep. Next morning, he comes to me. He hugs and kisses me. "I'm sorry, but I didn't know what to say. I don't know what to tell you. The only thing I can say is that I love you and you can count on me."

Ramón says that the support of his family and children gave him courage to face HIV and AIDS. "I got to love life even more." But Ramón did not tell his children about his homosexuality—only about having HIV.

Heriberto faced a similar situation. He simultaneously acknowledged his HIV status and his homosexuality while talking to his parents. As with Ramón, Heriberto looked for a support group immediately after he tested HIV positive in Brazil. Heriberto did not feel comfortable during his initial visit. The second time, however, things clicked. "It felt like home. It was very little, a very small group. We stuck together for many years."

After participating in the group, Heriberto told his sisters that he had HIV. He did not want to tell his parents. He felt it would be difficult to talk to them about his status because of the stigma surrounding HIV. He also worried because they did not know about his homosexuality. But he was forced to tell them when he fell ill with tuberculosis and was hospitalized. Heriberto thought he was going to die:

> My mother was very angry. . . . And my father was very sad and understanding. But my mother was angry with the whole thing, 'cause with the HIV I was also saying, "Look, I'm gay, I'm homosexual." They had no idea.

Heriberto's mother, unlike others discussed before, was not initially supportive. Both parents provided Heriberto with a home and an income to live on while he was ill. They also helped him move to Europe and, then, to the United States so Heriberto could have access to the latest medications to fight HIV.

Just as it happens when telling others about their sexual orientation, some of these activists use, explicitly or implicitly, their disclosure of HIV status to educate others. The education occurs to varying degrees. It may run the range from merely knowing someone with HIV or AIDS, to getting into the numerous details about medicines, HIV viral loads and T-cells. Actually, most of these activists by the nature of their activism are constantly educating others.

When Jack became HIV positive, he also made himself what he refers to as an "HIV-positive poster child." He was doing a college internship with a local AIDS organization, when the organization was looking for an HIV-positive person to participate in a panel. He volunteered to do it and, in doing so, began his career as activist:

> When I first came out, I was like this HIV-positive poster child. I was young, and nobody was speaking in [my hometown] about being positive.
>
> So, people started taking notice of this young Latino boy that was positive and wasn't afraid to say he was. Any opportunity that presented itself, I was on it, "I'll do it."

Jack's account is a fair example among these activists of the type of educational work that they do. They are constantly educating the public. They are likewise educating their families, significant others, and close friends. Frequently, the lack of information about HIV and AIDS leads to unfounded concerns by others. Thus, some of these activists try to keep their love ones informed to avoid unnecessary worries, as Brian explains in the next excerpt:

> I did tell my mom and my family about [my HIV status]. When it comes to people that are a part of my life. I need to be open about everything. Sometimes that's good; sometimes that's not good. I think it's for the best, in the long run anyway.
>
> I still find that I can't tell my mom a lot of things because she becomes too emotionally upset and it's not good for her. With my sister, it is a bit different. I've sent her tons of information. This is what HIV is, this is what HIV is not, this is what AIDS is, this is what AIDS is not, this is where I'm at. They're informed, because I've informed them. I don't want them having all these worries.

All but a couple of these activists are open about their HIV or AIDS status. They are open to their close friends, boyfriends, partners, and perhaps most important and difficult, to their families. The exceptions are with the latter, as a couple of men have not informed their families that they have HIV. Notably, in some instances, the disclosure to families was not voluntary, as some of these activists became so ill that their families were informed by either friends or doctors. Likewise, most of them have the support of their immediate families, friends, boyfriends, and partners. And this is perhaps one of the major reasons they are still alive, living a relatively healthy life and involved in social and political affairs. The support of their families, *compañeros*, boyfriends, and partners has made them resilient.

Although praise for the work of social support groups is almost unanimous, there are caveats in what these groups can do and what they have been able to do. Carmen, who lives in San Francisco, criticizes such groups for being just another place to meet sexual partners. She explains that they lack any ability to deal with the basic concerns of participants. In speaking of group meetings, she says, "There is always the same thing. Only talking about *cogederas* [sex and nonsense]. 'When was your first time?' 'Who fucked you the first time?' 'Are you in love?'" She further elaborates:

> In the group I was in, there was a *cogedera*. Instead, why don't they ask, "Do you have a place to live?" "Do you have food?" "You want to study but you can't? We'll help you get in school." To support us is to say, "Hey, Joe, you just got here from Nicaragua and you don't know any English? First, we got to teach you English so you can make it in this country and people don't take advantage of you." That's to be brothers, not *mariconadas* [fag things].

Although Carmen's view might not be generalizable, I can corroborate some of the points that she raises based on my own experience with HIV and AIDS groups and organizations in the United States and Mexico. Regardless of their intentions, many men meet boyfriends and sexual partners in these support groups. It would be expected for this to occur as the support groups provide one of the few opportunities for gay men and transgender persons to socialize. Moreover, in the tradition of U.S. psychology, social support groups are not designed to address people's basic life necessities, such as education and employment. They are about dealing with people's concerns through dialogue.

In addition, these types of groups, at least those related to HIV and AIDS, are usually underfunded and cannot maintain professional staff or address participants' basic needs (without becoming social service agencies).

Changing the Self

The proximity of death and the recognition of one's mortality that come with HIV and AIDS threaten the sense of security and prompt a reevaluation of one's life. While they do not change the core of the self, certain aspects of one's life become a priority. Some qualities of the self come to the foreground, while others recede to the background. That is, the life perspective is changed. HIV and AIDS also bring a sense of urgency to life; an exigency to the plans and the dreams. Plans, dreams, and reconciliations can not be postponed until tomorrow or for better circumstances. This is a cultural narrative about confronting mortality that helps one face death and move on with living.

Almost any epidemic of the magnitude of AIDS results in profound changes in societies. AIDS, in particular, changed the place of homosexuality in the social landscape, for both insiders and outsiders. The dominant medical and societal discourse around HIV and AIDS attacked sexual freedom, that is, the freedom from the constraint of moral Christian values, such as heterosexuality and monogamy. For example, the AIDS epidemic led officials in San Francisco to close the widely popular bathhouses, which were the spaces in which some sexual freedom is enacted, albeit in an enclosed area. One witness, Simon, describes this social and personal transformation:

> They closed the bathhouses. That impacted my sexual life! For me, the best thing about being gay was the bathhouses. I wouldn't care if they were to close the bars. For me, it's about the sex . . . getting into a bathhouse and seeing a beautiful naked male body, the erect penis, the glances, the rush, and then the sex. I was addicted.
> And then we had to use condoms. It is not the same as before.

Some of these changes and their consequences have been reversed after two decades. Some bathhouses have reopened, sex clubs have flourished, and condoms are becoming less popular.

But at the personal level, at the core of the self, HIV and AIDS can bring more profound and lasting transformations than those at the societal level, particularly for those living with HIV/AIDS. In the 1980s and 1990s, mere diagnosis was tantamount to a death sentence. Hence, the transformation brought about by HIV was immediate and quite radical. As the medical treatment for HIV and AIDS improved since the turn of the millennium, the change of the self has become less radical than it was in the 1980s and 1990s. Still, an HIV diagnosis, along with exacting medical treatments and full-blown AIDS, can change almost anybody's sense of self.

Jack received HIV-positive tests results in 1992. But he believes that he actually became HIV positive in 1989. HIV, he says, gave him a strong desire to live and a sense of being in touch with the core of his own self, a state that he had not experienced before:

> I felt like, "Oh, shit!" At the time, AZT was on the market. But we still were dealing with the fear of dying. I wanted to live my life to the fullest. I wanted to make an impact in life, impact communities.
> I felt like HIV had really given me this, like, attunement to life that I had never had before. It gave me like a third eye. . . . I was very much in tune with my sorrow. I was very much in tune with the good and the bad in me. I was very much in tune with the capabilities that I had to do wrong, to do good, to be sad, to let my trials and tribulations teach me.

The change that Jack talks about it is not that of becoming a new or different person. It is about continuing to be himself but in a more true manner than before; being in tune with his own self, as he would put it. This means accepting and recognizing who he was, including his new HIV status. It also implies living life fully, which for him means speaking out and becoming actively involved in the AIDS movement to help change the course of the epidemic.

Like Jack, Ramón says that "the virus" has taught him about life, has helped him live a fuller life than before, and forced him to be himself:

> It made me look at myself and [my] love life. Despite all the bad stuff, the virus has taught me beautiful things, like meeting so many people and sharing with so many others.
>
> The virus taught me to live, to see life in a different manner, like getting involved with other people. I have learned to accept myself and live true to myself, without worrying about what others would say.

HIV has brought significant changes in Ramón's life and self-concept. After Ramón learned that he was HIV positive and attended a support group, he disclosed to his family that he had HIV. As a result of HIV, he also became an activist along with other HIV-positive people. Ramón has thus come to live a fuller and public life as a person living with HIV. His core has not changed; rather, only the manner in which he relates with others and the way in which he sees life have changed.

In San Francisco, Renato expresses a similar sentiment, but his narrative of change focuses on using the time that is left to its fullest:

> When I became HIV positive, of course, part of me lost control. Mentally, I was sure—I was twenty-three—and I knew I was never going to make it to thirty. So I decided I had to do everything that I wanted to do in my life. I learned French, I got certified in scuba diving, I joined a gym. I started going back to Puerto Rico all the time. I spent a lot more time with my friends and developing the close friendships, and I got a boyfriend who was also HIV positive.
>
> It has been a blessing. Everyone that I knew from that era, when I was twenty-three, is dead. I feel an incredible gift that I'm alive.
>
> It made me much more aware of the beauty of living. . . . My spiritual life has really brought me a lot closer at a spiritual level than I think I had been before. My consciousness for social justice I think is influenced by HIV so much and all the things that I'm doing are really a product of HIV.

Thus, the majority of *compañeros* living with HIV and AIDS claim that the virus, while transforming their lives, has not fundamentally altered them as people. The forty-year-old Alfonso states, "it changed the way I live, not my life." They also maintain that HIV and AIDS have offered them an opportunity and a lesson. Alfonso explains, "it has not been a curse, as I first thought, but a blessing." The lesson is that one can not live guided by others' rules and expectations, putting them before one's own wishes. The opportunity is to be true to oneself and attempt to realize one's dreams. Furthermore, the change these activists speak about is one of perspectives. HIV and AIDS have made many of these activists see life through spiritual and religious eyes.

Abraham tells a somewhat different story and a different type of change. He was raised going back and forth between New York City and Puerto Rico and at the age of seventeen found out he was HIV positive. HIV actually changed his sense of self. He ceased to be one person and became another:

> It was really hard, and I remember at that point I was no longer a teenager. That's when I was really pushed into adulthood, because I had to deal with death. And I remember that from that point on everything was weird, it was never the same.
>
> I just think that being HIV positive puts this whole thing in perspective. I'm going to die. I don't know how long I have to live, so I don't have to care about what my family thinks anymore. I see myself eventually moving to New York, but I don't want to feel like my dreams are going to be stopped.

Unlike other activists, Abraham states that HIV changed him. It changed not only his way of living, but who he is. The virus, he says, put an end to his teenhood and forced him to become an adult. Seeing himself at the point of dying and, after surviving that experience, dealing with HIV altered his life, making him an adult. After HIV, he could no longer act as if he were unaware of his mortality. He now knows that he might die, maybe not soon, but that simple realization has made him love life and has motivated him to pursue his dreams.

Finally, there are those who claim that HIV neither transformed them nor brought any positive changes to their lives. Mateo, who lives in Chicago, says that being HIV positive has not had any impact on his life: "I accept and live my condition as an HIV-positive person. It hasn't changed me in any way." Heriberto, who emigrated from Brazil and lives in San Francisco, ponders what his life would have been like without HIV:

> Sometimes I'm curious. Would my life be different, if I wasn't HIV positive? That's one thing I think I'll never have the answer for. Maybe if I wasn't HIV positive, I would be still living in Brazil. I would have finished my college.
>
> I had to sacrifice myself a little bit in a way. For example, I think the best place for somebody to be in is his own country, his own culture. But now, because

I left Brazil so long ago, it's hard to go back, but on the other hand, I wish I could be there, still.

The experience of HIV and AIDS changed the lives of most of these activists. The transformations these activists have experienced at the personal level can be categorized as alterations (McAdam 1989; Ramirez-Valles 1999; Travisano 1981). Alterations are usually defined vis-à-vis conversions. The latter refers to profound changes of the self, usually involving the adoption of a new identity. Alterations entail subtle changes within the same self-identity. Although one could argue that calling oneself "HIV-positive" or "poz" might imply a new identity, the narratives of these activists show that being HIV positive is for the most part incorporated into the existing self. That is, the changes brought about by HIV and AIDS only modify the already-available identity, as either Latino, gay man, or transgender. We return to this theme of alterations in chapter 7.

Still, as with most changes, some behaviors and values are replaced by new ones. In the case of HIV/AIDS, we learned that these activists got close to their sense of themselves; came to appreciate their health, their loved ones, their relationships with others, and their lives in a new and revitalized way; realized the need to get involved in community affairs; and developed a more in-depth religious and spiritual perspective than they had before. Their stories, thus, speak of positive changes in the face of HIV and AIDS.

Implicit in the changes these activists have undergone, thus, there is a moral lesson. This is most clearly seen in Jimmy's reflection:

> Life's beatings have made me mature. Life has taught me many things; things that I ignored and didn't know their consequences. Now, I think about the consequences of my acts before I do anything. For example, if I begin smoking. What consequences will it have? I'll damage the liver, on top of the damage created by the meds. So, it doesn't make sense to smoke.

The lesson is one of personal responsibility and is fueled by the stigma toward HIV and AIDS. One is responsible for what happens to one's self in this life. One is responsible for the misfortunes and pain encountered. If only one were to act according to the norms enacted, say, by medicine and Roman Catholicism, and the potential consequences of one's acts, the self would be free of suffering, of HIV, and shame.

HIV and AIDS are just two defining events in the lives of these men. They are illuminating destinations along the course of a much longer journey in their lives. They are one of the many changes that these activists have encountered, and will encounter, in the course of their lives. Their participation in AIDS and LGBT organizations, as we see in the next two chapters, is another leg in the journey that will transform their lives. Yet, this particular situation, HIV and AIDS, is especially enlightening because it is closely tied to the very existence of these participants, as human beings and as gay and bisexual men and transgender persons.

These *compañeros* joined the AIDS movement because of their personal experiences with HIV and AIDS. They came to see the epidemic from the inside. They felt and saw the paucity of health-care services and the ineffectiveness of prevention efforts. They also felt different: alienated, shameful, and guilty. But just as they did when creating their identities as gay men and transgender persons, they sought out and found others. As they joined support groups and community organizations, they found *compañeros*, who provided information, companionship, comfort, and a positive identity as people living with HIV or AIDS. Perhaps as important as that support, *compañeros* provided the space for them to become involved in HIV and AIDS affairs.

CHAPTER SIX

GETTING INVOLVED

Gerardo and Orlando, both from Chicago, were involved in the creation of two small, distinct organizations: a volunteer-based organization of Latino gay men and an organization dedicated to providing HIV education and prevention services for Latino and black gay and bisexual men. Gerardo and Orlando are both in their forties; they worked in the same city with different groups of men. Although they took different paths, the circumstances that led them to the creation of those organizations are quite alike and remarkably similar to the ones that led me to the AIDS movement.

In the late 1980s, when the AIDS epidemic and social movement were escalating, Gerardo was working in a social-services organization conducting programs related to substance abuse prevention. He was invited to attend a conference on Latino gay men in Chicago. There he found himself surrounded by Latinos, especially gay men, from major cities such as Los Angeles, San Francisco, and New York. He also saw many of his gay friends. Of this time, Gerardo says:

> All of us, who knew each other from different things, like the bars, were like "Oh my God, girl, how'you doing?" We were sitting outside and there were these guys from LA, from San Francisco, and two people from New York. They were talking about Chicago.

When visitors asked about the Latino gay organizations in Chicago, Gerardo and his friends could name Latino organizations and groups, but no Latino *and* gay. "Actually, there isn't a single one," Gerardo would reply.

The lack of Latino gay organizations bugged Gerardo for some time until he realized it represented an opportunity to form one. He knew a few other Latino gay men working in social services. They had attended the same conference. He himself had experience in nonprofit organizations and social services. He gathered his friends and launched the idea of the only organization for and by Latino gay men in the city:

> I kept thinking: "You know, I don't know why there isn't one." "I know all these great gay Latino guys, we could put an organization together. It's not that big of a deal. I worked in a not-for-profit, and I'm a director of programs. I know what it's like. I know what it takes."
>
> I started the organization along with three other friends of mine. We had brunch, and next thing we know, we were throwing out names and acronyms.

Looking for a space to hold meetings, Gerardo and his friends approached what Gerardo calls a "white" gay organization, which agreed. They set up a series of forums for Latino gay men. They also developed bylaws and formed a board of directors. Within two years the group became well-known among gay communities in Chicago, in spite of the fact that it lacked external funding and a space of its own. In those two years, according to Gerardo, the group struggled to form its own identity and to remain independent. Some of the men who joined the organization were more interested in socializing and meeting potential boyfriends and sexual partners than in working on the social and political issues facing Latino gay men. In addition, established gay organizations wanted to co-opt the group:

> First we had the parasites, the guys that were like, "I want to get some Latinos." Then, the white community, of course, was like, "Oh my God, a gay Latino group. We have to co-opt them right away." I had a huge fight with men of all colors.
>
> We had bylaws and we had a mission statement. We had real board meetings and, of course, the guys are like [yawning], bored. But we needed that structure; because the thing that has made other groups fail was that they were too social. I really wanted it to be a safe space so that anyone who came would know this is legitimate, this is a real organization. I had gone to other groups like, Men of All Colors and those were really hunting grounds, especially for white men who were looking for men of color. And still the overall leadership was white men.

The organization has remained independent, albeit with limited funding. In fact, it only obtained nonprofit status a few years ago. The organization has also maintained some distance from AIDS. Gerardo and other leaders have purposely rejected the temptation to get funding from AIDS sources, such as local and federal governments and private foundations.

This became evident to me when I first joined the organization in the late 1990s. I volunteered to cofacilitate a social group. Those attending the meetings did not want to talk about HIV or sexual risk behavior. That did not mean they were indifferent to those issues. Rather, it meant that HIV and sexual risk were not their main concerns, and they were tired of being lectured at and being seen only as a "population at risk." In the discussions, we would talk about HIV, our own fears, and about our health, but such topics did not define the agenda of those meetings.

Around the same time, and on the other side of town, Orlando was creating an AIDS organization. Unlike Gerardo, Orlando had already tested HIV positive; he was pursuing his graduate studies and was working on a needle-exchange program to prevent HIV. Orlando also had recently lost a close friend to AIDS. Two researchers from the university where he was studying approached him. They had obtained funding to do research on HIV on Latino and black homosexual men. They did not have direct access to such groups, however. One of the researchers contacted him:

> They wanted to look at some questions around minority gay men. She saw me in the health club and one day she came to me. She knew I worked for the needle exchange. She asked me: "Are you gay?" I said, "Yeah, can't you tell?" After joking around, she goes: "This guy I'm working with wants to do some research." I said, "Well, you know what, I'd be really interested in being part of it, because maybe it will allow me a chance to provide some services."
>
> I figured, OK, if you're going to get research, you're going to have to figure out a way to find these people. Maybe he can provide some money so I can get the people, and we can go out there and do some education.

Orlando agreed; along with the woman and another colleague, he formed a small organization to collect the data needed by the researcher and to provide prevention activities for Latino and Black gay men. Orlando adopted the community-organizing model from the needle-exchange program and applied it to gay men. The model, very much like the model I learned from the women's health organization in Mexico, relies on indigenous leaders to deliver health messages and services in their own communities.

Once the research project concluded, Orlando and his two colleagues wanted to continue providing HIV education. They wrote a grant proposal for the Chicago Department of Public Health to support the service mission of the organization. Orlando and colleagues were concerned mainly with HIV and AIDS. They did not care much about the sexual identity of the men they were working with. Whether those men identified themselves as gay, homosexual, transvestite, or bisexual did not matter for the purposes of the organization.

Orlando invited me to join the board of the organization in 1999. Unfortunately, the organization had to close down a couple of years later due to lack of funding. For Orlando, the creation of this organization was a type of calling. The year before university researchers approached him, Orlando had lost a friend to AIDS on the East Coast. At one point, Orlando had flown there to take care of him. "That was his way of telling me to get involved in this."

Gerardo, Orlando, and I belong to the same generation marred by AIDS. Our generation grew up during the nascent gay movement. As adults, we witnessed its change from avant-garde to moderate agenda and activism. We were in different social and geographical spaces (even though Gerardo and Orlando lived in the same city, their lives were taking place in different spaces). Through different paths, the three of us got involved in the AIDS and gay movements. Our paths, however, share common features that were crucial to our involvement. We were Latino and gay, had college degrees, and had earned moderate incomes. Most significant in our involvement was our work experience. The three of us worked in social service and health-related agencies. We had skills that were easily transferable to AIDS and gay-related issues. We knew the "how-to." Also, our jobs and social networks exposed us to opportunities to get involved by way of volunteering and activism.

This path to activism is not very common among this group of activists, as can be seen in table 2 ("Through work" row). Yet it highlights factors crucial for involvement and the founding of grassroots groups, as exemplified by the first efforts of gay men in New York City and San Francisco to fight AIDS (Chambré 2006). These factors have to do with the ability to mobilize resources and include group membership, education, skills, experience, and social networks with similar resources. Individuals with such

Table 2. Frequency of Means of Community Involvement in HIV & AIDS Organizations in Chicago and San Francisco*

Means of Community Involvement	Chicago n (%) (n=40)	San Francisco n (%) (n=40)	Total n (%) (n=80)
Friends & relatives	8 (20)	14 (35)	22 (28)
Accessing services	13 (33)	8 (20)	21 (26)
Media	6 (15)	11 (28)	17 (21)
School & university	7 (18)	6 (15)	13 (16)
Paid job	10 (25)	0	10 (13)
Through work	5 (13)	4 (10)	9 (11)
Through a partner	4 (10)	3 (8)	7 (9)
Church	1 (3)	3 (8)	4 (5)
Other**	1 (3)	3 (5)	4 (5)

*Participants could report more than one means of involvement.

**"Other" refers to means of involvement that were mentioned infrequently by participants: through flyers, court, and walk-in.

resources, such as Gerardo, are able to initiate community organization. They are also likely to be invited to join, as was Orlando.

In this chapter I trace the paths to activism and volunteerism. I address the question of how these activists actually became part of the AIDS and gay movements. My analysis is informed by the literature on recruitment in social movements (Cable 1992; Hunt et al. 1994; Simon et al. 2000), which underlines the social nature of getting involved. Participation is shaped by the social location of individuals (e.g., social class, ethnicity, identity) and by what Snow and colleagues refer to as the frame alignment process (1980, 1986). This is defined as an interactive phenomenon by which individuals' beliefs, grievances, and actions are linked to the agenda of a social movement organization (Snow et al. 1986).

The frame alignment is achieved as individuals are recruited into organizations. The recruitment process starts when a contact is established with a potential participant (Snow et al. 1980). This usually takes place through social networks. At this point, potential members are provided with information about the organization and, or, its activities. Then, prospective participants evaluate their availability in terms of alternative commitments and possible conflict with their own norms and social networks (Cable 1992; Snow et al. 1980). If individuals are available, they are offered an invitation not to actually join, but to participate in an activity or a meeting so they can interact with other members and get to know the organization. It is here where participants form their motives to join and begin to align them with the organization's agenda.

Tables 2 through 5 summarize the basic features of this process of involvement. Table 2 lists by city the means by which *compañeros* become involved. Friends and relatives are the most commonly reported means of involvement, followed by LGBT or AIDS agencies, and media. The categories

Table 3. Frequency of Types of Organizations Reported for Community Involvement by City*

Organization Type	Chicago (n=40)	San Francisco (n=40)	Total (n=80)
HIV & AIDS	34	51	85
Lesbian, Gay, Bisexual, Transgender	32	21	53
Other**	11	13	25

*Participants could have reported either, or both, categories.

**"Other" organizations include hospice for the terminally ill, drug and rehabilitation clinics and programs, arts organizations, and college organizations.

Table 4. Frequency of Involvement by Organization Type and City*

Chicago		San Francisco	
LGBT CBOs**	Frequency	LGBT CBOs	Frequency
ALMA	9	*AGUILAS–El Ambiente*	9
Howard Brown Health Center	6	Queens of color	3
Horizons	5	Larkin Street Youth Center	2
En la Vida Magazine	4	Coalition of gay, bi, trans, Concerns	2
Gay Pride Parade	3	Gay Pride Parade	1
Amigas Latinas	1	GLAAD	1
Gay/Lesbians Straight Club	1	Lyric	1
Lion's Pride	1	*Quelaco*	1
Queer Newspaper**	1	Sentinel Newspaper	1
Talents of IL Transgender	1		
HIV/AIDS CBOs		**HIV/AIDS CBOs**	
Minority Outreach Intervention Project	5	San Francisco AIDS Foundation	10
CALOR	4	*Instituto Familiar de la Raza/Proyecto Mano a Mano*	5
Project Vida	4	Open Hand	5
AIDS Walk	3	Shanti	5
Open Hand	3	*Projecto contra SIDA por VIDA*	4
Test Positive Aware Network	3	AIDS Walk	3
Vida/SIDA	3	Under One Roof	3
AIDS Foundation of Chicago	2	Stop AIDS Project	2
Stop AIDS Chicago	2	AIDS Emergency Fund	1
AIDS Ministry	1	AIDS Project of the East Bay	1
Bonaventure House	1	AIDS Recycling Program	1
ERIE Family Health Center	1	AIDS Ride	1
Hispanic AIDS Network	1	ARIS (AIDS research)	1
HOLAA	1	Body Positive SIDA Ahora	1
		Care Council	1
		Discover Group	1
		Latino AIDS Project	1
		Mission Neighborhood Health Center/Hermanos de Luna y Sol	1
		Positive Resource Center	1
		POZ Magazine	1
		RACORSE (Medical equipments recycling org.)	1
		UCSF AIDS Health Project	1

*Note: Participants could have volunteered at more than one organization. Italicized organizations are predominantly or exclusively Latino/a.

**CBO = Community-based organization.

***Name of the newspaper was not specified.

Table 5. Frequencies of Community Involvement Activities in Chicago and San Francisco*

Community Involvement Activities	Chicago n (%) (n=40)	San Francisco n (%) (n=40)	Total n (%) (n=80)
Outreach	17 (43)	18 (45)	35 (44)
Education	14 (35)	15 (38)	29 (36)
Help to HIV+ & PWAs	13 (32)	16 (40)	29 (36)
General help	10 (25)	16 (40)	26 (33)
Office help	7 (18)	18 (45)	25 (31)
Board memberships	13 (32)	9 (23)	22 (28)
Coordinating/organizing events	8 (20)	10 (25)	18 (23)
Group facilitator/coordinator	12 (30)	5 (13)	17 (21)
Fund-raising	9 (23)	6 (15)	15 (19)
Protests, marches, demonstrations & rallies	6 (15)	5 (13)	11 (14)
Founding an organization	6 (15)	2 (5)	8 (10)
Hotline operator	3 (8)	5 (13)	8 (10)
Lobbying	2 (5)	1 (3)	3 (4)
Other**	4 (10)	1 (3)	5 (6)

*Participants could report more than one activity.
**"Other" refers to activities that were mentioned infrequently by participants, e.g., development of HIV resource room, helped at a conference, recycled unused HIV medicine to Latin America, administered HIV tests, and participated in HIV research.

represented here are not mutually exclusive; one can be recruited by several means to join different organizations at different times.

Table 3 presents the distribution of the types of organizations (e.g., LGBT and AIDS) in which these activists have been involved. This table is followed by a distribution of the actual organizations in which these activists have participated in each city (table 4).

Finally, table 5 summarizes activities reported by these activists. The most common activities include outreach (e.g., distributing education materials and condoms), education, helping people living with HIV and AIDS, and general help. Notably, only a small number of activists report participating in protests, marches, and rallies. While it is difficult to draw solid conclusions from these data, I think the activities are a reflection of the current state of the AIDS and gay movements. Few groups are involved in direct action, which includes rallies and demonstrations (ACT UP is one of the groups that does use direct action). Most of the actions of those movements have been institutionalized. They have been converted into social services and nonprofit organizations. Thus, we see many volunteers involved in outreach, education, and providing general help. The activities also reflect cohort and generational effects. The younger group of activists (e.g., 18 to

30 years old) joined the AIDS and gay movements when they were already institutionalized; whereas the older group witnessed the rising of the gay and AIDS movements, when protests and rallies were more common.

Friends and Family

Scholars working on volunteerism and social movements have emphasized social networks as the predominant recruitment sources. Friends, *compañeros,* and relatives, all part of our social networks, invite us to organizations and volunteer activities. That is part of the social support they provide. They open new opportunities and new roads for us.

Eduardo, for example, was invited to an AIDS Walk by his friend and neighbor. Eduardo had left his hometown in Texas behind. He had never been involved in either LGBT or AIDS issues, despite being openly gay and living with his partner. His neighbor, a woman, was the coordinator for the local AIDS Walk in Southern California. When she invited Eduardo to join, he thought it would be a good opportunity to meet other people and "give back to the community." Eduardo recalls:

> Well, the first time I volunteered for HIV and AIDS was when I was living with my partner. My next-door neighbor was the coordinator of the AIDS Walk, and she asked me: "Do you want to volunteer?" I said, "Sure."
>
> She said, "I think you'd have more fun if you actually helped put it together. I think you would enjoy it more. Why don't you just come to an orientation and see what you think." One of the issues was that she was my neighbor, and then I thought it would be an interesting way to meet people. I wanted to give back to the community, and that was an easy way to do it.
>
> I went to orientation, talked about what the positions were. I helped put the walk together. I met a lot of different people. It was a lot of fun.

In Eduardo's recollection of events, we see how the bond between friends can be the reason for accepting such an invitation. We also appreciate the construction of motives. In Eduardo's account, it is made implicit that the AIDS Walk is a worthwhile cause. There is no need to explain its purpose. What is made explicit is the "fun" aspect of volunteering as a motive to participate. Eduardo is invited. He subsequently forms his own motives, in order to meet others and give back to the community. Moreover, Eduardo was invited not to join but to attend an orientation session as an opportunity for him to get to know the organization and the activities. Before we join, we are usually invited to a meeting or orientation.

The process of being recruited by an organization and constructing motives to get involved is also evident in Sergio's experiences in Chicago. He is twenty-six years old and completed one year of graduate school. His cousin, who is also gay, recruited Sergio to join the Latino gay organization. The cousin, who was volunteering in the same organization, was trying to create a website for the organization but had limited expertise in using the needed software. He called Sergio for help because of his skills in software and information technology. Subsequently, Sergio received a call from the organization's director, inviting him to join:

> Then [the director] called. "You know, we're having a meeting on such and such a day. Would you like to come?" I said, "Sure." So I went and it was fun.
> He called me a few days later and asked me if I would help him out, because he needed a secretary. "Sure, why not?" It'll give me something to do, keep me busy, and I can meet people.

Like Eduardo, Sergio was first invited to attend an event, which served as an introduction to the organization and to its volunteers. In the process, Sergio formed his reasons and motivations for participating. In this case, volunteering would be a good use of his leisure time and would provide him the opportunity to be around peers.

Manuel joined the same organization via a member friend. Manuel, a Mexican immigrant, is fifty-four years old and has HIV. A friend invited him to one of the brunches hosted by the gay group. He attended the brunch and saw that his knowledge of accounting and finances would enable him to contribute to the organization. "I saw how they were fumbling and had stumbling blocks in growth due to the fact that they had very little business knowledge."

Manuel subsequently became a volunteer. He helped the organization with financial reporting and bookkeeping. He also helped draft an application and secure a grant. He assisted the organization with writing and budgeting.

Manuel's involvement began in the late 1960s, while he was in college. Within the context of student and gay movements, his story illustrates how we also get involved with friends. While friends recruit, they also join in their roles as *compañeros*. We get involved with our friends and *compañeros*:

> Once I got to college, it was such a fast-paced kind of thing. A friend of mine and I began the gay social club. He and I were the only members. It was around the Vietnam War and all of the turbulence.
> They gave us one room and then we got a record player and we started playing records. We said, "This is the gay club," like the Spanish club, and people would go by and kind of looked at us as if we were from the moon.

Then we started looking at what it was to be gay. We started going to the library and getting Oscar Wilde books. At that time, Roosevelt University had about fifteen books on homosexuality, and so we'd get them out and put them on top of our desk. A big book, this big, with the word "Homosexuality." It was that kind of boldness just to have the back of a book say "homosexuality," with pictures of who knows what.

In the early 1970s, Manuel used to perform in drag shows in a Latino gay bar. When the Howard Brown Health Center opened its doors, it became the first health clinic for the LGBT community in the city. Manuel and his friends lent their artistic skills in order to raise funds:

> In the mid '70s, there was a well-known Latino bar on the corner of Halsted and Schubert called El Dorado. It was mostly for Latino gay people. Howard Brown had just opened its office across the street. At that time, it was just for checking for lice, gonorrhea, and syphilis. Most of the people that were there were college graduates, white guys, young, good-looking. At the beginning, it was a nice place to meet somebody to date. It was the first feeling of going into an all-gay environment.

At the clinic, Manuel was invited to volunteer. He and a couple of friends began staging drag shows as fund-raising events. "We could dress in drag at a drop of a hat," he recollects. In the early 2000s, Manuel got involved with the Latino gay men organization and eventually joined its board of directors. He also participated in an AIDS organization that serves Latino and Black gay men.

When I met our next activist, Bernardo, in 2002, he was a volunteer and on the board of an AIDS organization in San Francisco. At that time he was thirty-nine years old and had recently returned to the Bay Area after three years in Southern California. A friend recruited him to the board of directors. Bernardo explains that his current position is more about management than activism. He did have some volunteer experience prior to his current affiliation with another AIDS organization:

> I wanted to do something to help the gay community. . . . Stop AIDS Project had a big sign that said, "We need volunteers." So I went there and they were doing outreach. That's what they needed me for.

Bernardo is HIV negative, has a successful career in private industry, and enjoys a comfortable life that gives him status among other volunteers. Bernardo was not recruited for his first volunteer experience. Nor was he looking for services. By his account, he walked into the office looking for an opportunity to help the gay community. Although as a shy person he was hesitant about a job that required an outgoing and assertive personality, he became involved in outreach work. He also asked to participate in other activities, and did some work on a couple of fund-raising events.

Following the AIDS Project, Bernardo provided support for people living with AIDS in San Francisco. He remembers a particular client he assisted at home who was seriously ill and suffered from paranoia. The client eventually went to a hospice. After that, Bernardo moved out of the Bay Area. Three years later, he returned and became part of the board of directors for the AIDS organization.

I close this section by presenting two examples of recruitment by relatives from activists in San Francisco. In the first one, Angelica became connected with an organization through her sister. Angelica was in high school in Southern California when her sister told her about a theater group called Drama Diva. Her sister knew the director of the organization, which involved queer youths of color in all aspects of theater production using the youths' own life experiences and stories. Angelica found herself as a transgender person through Drama Diva and became involved in other LGBT and AIDS organizations.

In the second case, Mario's community involvement began with his son, who is gay. Mario is fifty years old and was married in his home country of El Salvador. His son invited him to join a group that was one of the pillars of the Latino gay community in San Francisco. Mario had come to the United States with his wife and children from Central America. After he divorced his wife, it took him several years to feel comfortable with his and his son's sexuality and identity as gay men:

> My son told me that it was a very nice program. He asked me if I wanted to go, but at first I said no. Back then I was dealing with many issues in my mind. He then asked me to go with him, together the two of us. So we tried it out.

Since then, Mario has volunteered in two other organizations, including Shanti, an AIDS organization.

Accessing Services

A significant number of *compañeros* became active in the AIDS and gay movement as a result of approaching organizations searching for social services. They first were "clients," in the language of many of these organizations. Afterward, they became volunteers and activists. The transformation from client to volunteer or activist is partly due to reciprocity. Recipients of services frequently feel obligated to work on behalf of the organization, because of the benefits they have received from the organization or because they do not want to be passive recipients of services. They want to feel they have worked for the benefits they obtain.

Two types of services are notable here: those related to LGBT issues and those related to HIV and AIDS. The first type is usually accessed when individuals are in the process of defining their sexual or gender identity. The second occurs when individuals have been diagnosed with HIV or AIDS.

Ramón tested HIV positive in 1990. In search of a support group a year later, he joined an AIDS organization in Chicago. After a year, when the group disbanded, Ramón and a couple of *compañeros* contacted another organization to continue the group and recruit more participants:

> After about a year of being in the group, which was founded by six people from different organizations, it fell apart.
>
> The organization had a small newspaper and they offered to run a notice for us about the group. They also offered a space for the group to meet. Back then we'd meet on Saturdays. And little by little, we became part of their organization.

In San Francisco, Alfonso followed a similar path. He migrated to the city in search of HIV treatments, when he learned that he was HIV positive in Mexico City. After knocking on several doors, he found a health clinic where people spoke Spanish, and through the clinic he secured access to treatment and other services, such as housing. With his limited English, he was having trouble finding information and resources. At the health clinic, he learned that the AIDS Foundation was looking for Spanish-speaking volunteers for the AIDS hotline. He found at the foundation the resources and information he was seeking. He likewise found the opportunity to help others:

> I volunteered for two years. It was a very beautiful experience. There I realized that many people had no access to information. All the volunteers shared and helped each other.

Alfonso does not volunteer for the hotline anymore. At the time of our conversation, he was serving in the San Francisco AIDS Care Council. The council is in charge of planning and overseeing AIDS funding and services.

Carmen also briefly volunteered for an AIDS hotline in San Francisco. She explains:

> I did it because I have AIDS and the desire to help others avoid AIDS, and also because of the alarming AIDS statistics in the Latino community. I got involved in the hotline because actually I was a client and there was a Latino group. There I met a few people and then I told them I also wanted to serve. Then I got trained.

Fabian's story provides a good example of how people become involved via services provided by LGBT organizations. At the time of his interview for this study, Fabian was volunteering for the Latino gay organization in Chicago. He was doing the same work I did a few years ago, facilitating the discussion group. But his first volunteer experience was with Horizons (now the Center on Halsted), the main LGBT organization in Chicago.

If you recall, Fabian came to the United States from Mexico with his wife. As he became conflicted about the gay life he had discovered in Chicago and his marriage, Fabian called the Horizons hotline. "I called when I came out of the closet . . . they helped me a lot." He received training to work on the hotline and volunteered for a few months. While working at the hotline, he learned about the Latino gay organization and its discussion group. He began attending the meetings. Five months later, one of the group facilitators quit, and Fabian was asked to facilitate the group. He was invited to facilitate largely because of the fact that he is a little older (in his midthirties) than most attendees, who are in their early twenties. Furthermore, he has a college degree, is bilingual, and is articulate.

The proliferation of social services for AIDS has opened opportunities for large sectors of the LGBT communities to become actively involved in their communities' affairs. This is where we see one of the unintended consequences of the AIDS epidemic and the institutionalization of the movement it sparked. While they created spaces for gay men to get involved and in the process find *compañeros,* a social-services approach dominates the current efforts rather than a social-change model.

Media

I moved to Chicago in 1997. One of the first habits I developed was to look for printed gay and Latino media. Every week, I would go to a coffee shop or a bookstore to check out the latest papers and magazines such as *En La Vida, Windy City Times,* and *Gay Chicago.* I would do the same in San Francisco, since my first visit in 1992. Reading these publications helped me get acquainted with local events and characters. That is how I learned about ALMA (Association of Latino Men for Action), among other gay, AIDS, and Latino organizations. I called ALMA and asked for information about their events. My intention was twofold. First, I wanted to meet other Latinos. I was eager to meet *compañeros.* Second, I wanted to learn about Latino gay organizations, volunteers, and activists. I began attending ALMA Sunday brunches and discussion groups. Then, I became a volunteer facilitator for the discussion group.

One of these activists, Pedro, had a similar experience. When he moved to Chicago, he had difficulty finding peers. He was in his late twenties and had attended graduate school. He could not find what he calls "other professional Latinos" like himself. He had white friends but not Latinos, "Back then I didn't know a lot of Latinos, and I wanted to start having friends," he says. "Our culture is very different." Through *En La Vida,* the only publication in Spanish for Latino LGBT audiences in Chicago, he learned about ALMA:

> I had gone out one time and I picked up an *En La Vida* and I found that number [ALMA], so I called. The first person that answered my call was this queeny guy, who is my friend now. He called me back right away. I thought he was a very cool person.
>
> He told me about the groups that they had. The next week, I went to one of the groups. It was just a lot of fun. Back then, they had a group that was called OYE for people that were coming out. I was beyond that point, but I still kept going to the group because I related to other Latino guys.

A significant number of the activists I talked with have used the media in the same manner. They have mostly looked in printed media and on the internet for opportunities to get involved. Some of these activists did not have any previous experience as either volunteers or activists before searching for opportunities in the media. Almost all of them, however, showed the initiative to seek out organizations that would enable them to get involved.

In San Francisco, Hernan went through the same process as Pedro and me. In 1982, he moved back to the Bay Area after being in a long-term relationship elsewhere. He did not know anybody in the area. As a result, he sought out opportunities to get involved and meet other gay and Latino men:

> I wanted to do something. I felt like I needed to do something. I tried to volunteer for a mental health agency, but they wanted me to do mostly clerical work. I got bored and I decided that I didn't want to do it anymore.
>
> There was this social worker who was organizing a gay Latino men's group. I saw it in the paper; I think it was in the *Gay Times.* I signed up. We were talking about things like what's it like being gay, what's it like being Latino, and how are you dealing with the issues around HIV.

For the *Sentinel,* a LGBT publication, Hernan and the social worker organizing the group wrote an article about being gay and Latino in San Francisco. Of the article Hernan says: "We were talking about the importance of developing a distinct culture. A distinct culture within the gay community; a gay Latino community." Hernan then enrolled in graduate school and stopped attending groups and volunteering. After graduating, he decided to get involved again. As he had done before, he searched for organizations in the *Gay Times.* He called several organizations and ended up volunteering at Aguilas, a Latino gay men's group.

An activist from Chicago, Ariel began his career as a volunteer also through a LGBT publication. In the early 1990s, Ariel was in the process of creating his own identity and left his Jehovah's Witnesses church, where he was an elder. He would read all the gay publications in town and found that Howard Brown Health Center, the largest LGBT clinic in the Midwest, was looking for volunteers. He started distributing meals for people living with AIDS. He eventually volunteered for other organizations until he returned to school.

After leaving college, Ariel went on to help create groups for queer youths in Chicago suburbs. He and a group of friends saw a need for a space for LGBT youths. Among the members of the group were a physician, a lawyer, a professor, and a student, with Ariel the only nonwhite gay man. The group created a nonprofit organization, and by 2002 the organization had created five other groups in the suburbs of Chicago. The organization had also received a sizable grant to conduct HIV prevention among youth.

Isidro came across ACT UP at a point in his life when he was forming his identity as a gay man. Before going to his first ACT UP meeting in San Francisco, he had attended a Coming Out event organized by ACT UP:

> I think as part of my coming-out process and trying to find myself, I joined ACT UP. In all honesty, the reason I joined was because there was a picture in the paper and I was like: "That guy's cute!" In my second meeting, all made sense to me: disobedience and activism. At that second meeting, they needed a secretary and I raised my hand. I was immediately in the thick of things.

School and University

Student life offers opportunities to explore oneself and get involved in a variety of groups. In stories such as Manuel's, we have seen students take up gay and AIDS activism. As a student, one has the time and willingness to seek out peers, activities, and new experiences. One is likely to be open to new ideas, sensations, and endeavors. For most people, student life is a path to self-discovery, sexually and otherwise. Accordingly, one seeks out groups and peers for the purpose of discovering oneself and forming one's gender and ethnic identity.

In addition, schools furnish opportunities to get involved. Students have access to organizations, including LGBT groups. Frequently, they have to volunteer or provide services to nonprofit organizations within or outside of school in order to fulfill school requirements. Recently, with the increased acceptance (or tolerance) of gender nonconforming behavior, high schools are also offering queer youth opportunities to get involved.

Ignacio, for example, first became involved in LGBT and AIDS affairs in his high school in Chicago. In high school he joined a gay-straight alliance, a type of group that has become popular in the United States. For him, the group was something like a "gay club," which would conduct campaigns to promote both sexual and racial diversity and workshops. Ignacio subsequently came out as a gay man. He and his boyfriend would hold hands while walking in the school halls.

He was invited to join GLSEN, the local chapter of the Gay, Lesbian, and Straight Education Network. Now nineteen, Ignacio has participated in several summits as a member of this group. The organization uses these summits as a forum to discuss issues such as sexuality, religion, and same-sex marriage. He also has assisted in setting up press conferences.

When Ignacio joined the group, there were only three Latinos: Ignacio, his boyfriend, and a male friend. He continued in the group after he graduated from high school. He argues that his presence as a Latino man in the group is important:

> The gay community is very Eurocentric, like white America. Where are all the colored folk? When I go to events, many times I'm one of the few Latinos. It doesn't bother me, because I'm used to it. Sometimes I feel uncomfortable, 'cause like I'd even be eating and here I am, from the ghetto. I'd do my own thing and everyone is eating properly. I feel like that's a white thing.

When asked how and why he first got involved, however, Ignacio says that he has always been involved in various groups. For example, when he was twelve years old he joined the friends of the library volunteer group in his neighborhood:

> I called them: "I want to volunteer." They're like: "OK." So I'm like twelve years old and everyone is like thirty-plus. And here I am. I'm the cotreasurer. I've always just been involved like that. I like that.

One of the most involved activists in Chicago, Rigoberto also traces his activism to the gay-straight alliance at his university campus. Rigoberto did not think of himself as a gay man when he started college. When he first learned about the gay organization on campus, he was not sure what to make of it: "Initially when I went to school, I heard about a gay group and I thought 'Wow!' I never ventured to one of their meetings."

Two years later, when Rigoberto adopted a gay identity, he joined the group. For him, being gay and an activist were part of the same identity:

> When I first figured out that I was gay, I went to the Gerber/Hart Library [the LGBT library in Chicago]. I did as much reading as I could, and I just decided that if I'm going to be gay, I'm going to be involved.

Rigoberto was ready to join a gay organization: "I'm comfortable. I know who I am, I'm going to do it. And I just showed up." He saw a poster on campus and decided to become part of the gay and straight alliance. He went on to join a dozen other groups, including Queer Nation Chicago, ACT UP Chicago, ALMA, and Gay, Lesbian and Bisexual Veterans.

Alberto's story of community involvement begins in college, but he did not join a campus organization. He was, in part, recruited by a friend. As a student in San Francisco, he had a work-study assignment in the career counseling office. There he developed a friendship with one of the counselors, a Latino gay man. The counselor told him about Aguilas and invited him to one of its social events:

> He told me about this group called Aguilas, which I never heard of before. He said, "Do you want to go to a party?" I said, "Sure!" That's how he got me involved.

Alberto, who now is forty-seven years old, joined the group and eventually was invited to join the board of directors. He became the coordinator for social events.

Paid Job

For a few activists I talked to, community involvement is either a paid full-time job, an extension of their paid jobs, or is an outcome of their employment by an AIDS or LGBT agency. As I stated at the beginning of this chapter, this way of entry into the AIDS movement reflects the institutionalization of what once was a grassroots movement. The availability of funding and organizations working in the AIDS movement, including nonprofit and public agencies in the late 1980s, meant that many of those (unpaid) activists moved into paid positions. Some of those activists continued with activism, while others became service providers or advocates. As the institutionalization set in, entry into the AIDS movement by way of a paid position turned into a common pattern.

George, who lives in the Chicago suburbs, serves as a good example of an activist in the era of AIDS institutionalization. He emigrated to the United States from Mexico when he was in his twenties. His first job was in a grocery store. When he enrolled in a community college he got a part-time job in a self-service laundry where he met a *paisano* (fellow countryman), who was a regular customer. The *paisano* worked for a social services agency coordinating substance abuse treatment programs. One day, he told George that the agency had received a grant from the county to conduct an HIV prevention program for Latino gay men. The agency was looking for a coordinator and the *paisano* invited George to apply,

George did not think the job was for him. "I had my doubts," he says. In an attempt to persuade him, the *paisano* explained that he only needed to coordinate a group of friends and that the time was flexible. Because George was comfortable studying and working part-time, he initially declined to apply. The *paisano*, however, continued to insist over several months. George eventually changed his mind:

> "Well, let me see," I told him because he was very persistent. I had an interview. They explained the program and the details about HIV and AIDS prevention. I thought: "What if I get into this?" "What if I give it a try?" They told me I was to work part-time, with a flexible schedule, and that I could have the group meetings whenever it was convenient.

George accepted the position. As he learned about the job he found reasons to participate, most importantly, as he saw the reaction of the attendees during the first meetings:

> In our first meeting, we had a person from the Red Cross. It was a talk about HIV and AIDS. When the presentation was over, everybody was pale, very quiet, and scared.
> The second meeting was on Día de los Reyes [Epiphany]. We had a *rosca* [an oval sweet bread] and we had a presentation on testing and counseling, with a person from the health department. And again, everybody was so scared. There I saw the need. I told myself: "OK, it looks that there is a very important task for me to do here. Let's go on."

George found the reason to remain in the job and became deeply involved in the AIDS movement with Latino gay men. He saw a need for HIV prevention. He also realized that he had the basic skills required for the job. He enjoyed working with people and could relate to the men. "I have a mission," he thought. "Maybe God gave me this ability to communicate with others."

The position evolved into a full-time job. George says he usually works more than forty hours a week; accompanying men who want to get tested for HIV, visiting people living with HIV and AIDS, taking men on field trips, and collaborating with other organizations in the area sometimes requires sixty-hour workweeks.

One other activist, also from Chicago, tells a parallel story. Gregorio, is HIV positive and joined a support group for people living with HIV and AIDS in Chicago, guided by a *compañera*, who worked for a social-services agency. In a familiar process, Gregorio got a paid position in the organization to coordinate the support group. A couple of years later, he began coordinating two HIV programs for Latino men. He also was elected to the local HIV and AIDS prevention-planning group. Gregorio's commitment to AIDS has taken him across the country and even to Mexico, participating in forums and creating coalitions.

The fact that the activists I encountered in this category live in Chicago (see table 2) reveals little about differences between Chicago and San Francisco. We should not draw any generalizations. I created this category to reflect the primary means of entry into the AIDS movement. The categories do not necessarily reflect individuals' current positions. Actually, I found that in both cities, a good number of activists hold, or have held, paid jobs in either AIDS or gay organizations. We can conclude, however, that the boundaries between activism and paid work are blurred. Oftentimes, a paid position paves the way to a personal mission and a lifetime commitment.

Partners and Boyfriends

Before meeting his partner, Abel was not sympathetic of AIDS volunteers. Abel is thirty-two years old and immigrated from Mexico. He thought that people who were doing outreach work or participating in support groups did not have anything else to do with their lives. He thought many people volunteered to do these activities not to change the world, but to feel good about themselves.

All of that changed when he met his partner, who was an AIDS activist in Southern California and led a social group of Latino gay men and did outreach in bars, streets, and bathhouses. He joined his partner in some of those activities. His motives, however, were quite selfish. "At the beginning I helped him because I wanted him to finish quickly so that we could have more time together." His motives changed as he continued helping his partner. He got interested in learning about HIV and AIDS. His egocentrism turned into idealism: "thinking that giving information and condoms could help save lives and make a difference."

Abel's experience is not very common among this group of Latinos. Only a small group of them talked about becoming involved because or through their partners or boyfriends. And very few of them talked about joining a group or organization to meet potential boyfriends.

Church

The last category I discuss is people whose churches led them to the AIDS movement. Given the limited involvement with institutionalized religion among *compañeros,* only four among the eighty have taken this path to activism. I discuss two of them.

Renato, who is HIV positive, spends most of his free time in one of the United Church of Christ congregations in San Francisco, where he volunteers. He has been doing this for several years, and his work has reached a national presence within the church:

> I am an openly gay Latino [in the church], and there are not that many openly gay Latinos at a national level. I have participated in many different committees. I've also been on the planning committee for the national gathering.

Through the church, he got involved with political prisoners in Latin America. Also, he would visit a prison in the Bay Area almost every week. In doing so, he learned about the larger organizations doing work on behalf of political prisoners. He became interested in Cuba. This pursuit then led him to an AIDS-drugs recycling program:

> I started developing contacts in Cuba. I learned that the HIV situation was a crisis there. I learned that they were still doing monotherapy with AZT, which totally flipped me out. I decided that I would take a trip and bring donations. From a friend of a friend, I found out that there was a small church group in Havana giving out medications.

There are two principal ways these activists became involved: through their friends and relatives, and by accessing services. These two means are central to the AIDS movement and to movements around health issues in general. As with most social movements, recruitment is primarily driven by social networks. We first invite our friends and relatives to join. These are people with whom we share values and leisure activities and with whom we feel a mutual obligation. Then, we invite acquaintances and coworkers; those who are further removed from our intimate space. And we are also invited to join by friends and relatives.

Recruitment via accessing services is peculiar, I propose, to the AIDS movement and, to a large degree, to other health social movements. This echoes David Sills's classic argument that the illness experience is a fundamental piece of the process of getting involved (1957; see also Brown and Mikkelsen 1990). In this case, those affected, directly and indirectly, by HIV and AIDS, or the stigmatization of gender nonconforming behavior approach organizations and groups in search of resources to remedy or cope with the conditions. They then become involved either because they feel an obligation to give in return or because they acquire an awareness of the need to participate in the movement.

If we switch perspectives and look at AIDS and LGBT organizations, we see that the means utilized to recruit volunteers mirror the means described by volunteers and activists themselves (Ramirez-Valles and Brown 2003). In Chicago, for instance, word of mouth is by far the most commonly used recruitment method. This is followed by advertisements, referrals, community outreach, newsletters, flyers, collaboration with other agencies, schools and universities, and churches.

But the process of getting involved, or the recruitment process, is not a mechanical set of steps. From having a friend, being invited to an event, learning about the organization, and then to joining, there is a social and meaning-making process. In the interactions that take place during the recruitment process, we find, create, or reshape our motives to join. We align our motives to those of the organizations with which we become a part.

CHAPTER SEVEN

FINDING COMPAÑEROS

A few hours into our conversation and toward the end of the interview, I asked Humberto about his volunteer work: "What was important about working with other Latinos?" He answered:

> To have that sense of home again. That feeling of family. Knowing that I can walk into the room where there are Latinos I really know; that I don't feel this thing that I have to clam up.
>
> With *americanos* you always hold back, unless you know them a little bit better. But I've learned never let down my guard with *americanos*, white Americans. And no matter how friendly they are, no matter how good they are to you, there's always going to be *la diferencia*. Whether they want to admit to it or not.

Finding *compañeros* and a home is at the heart of community involvement. Our community involvement is about *compañeros* and creating a home as much as it is about making social change and helping others. This is the major consequence of getting involved. We connect with others, who in turn link us to the wider world. In doing so, we come to realize who we are and where we are.

Through getting involved we connect with others with whom we share an interest, an agenda, an identity, a common past, and *cariño* (affection). We also share a language, which means we share an implicit set of rules and norms about who we are and the Other (e.g., "the *americanos*"). That is, we connect with *compañeros*. They could be peers, friends, or colleagues. But *compañeros* are more than that. They are partners with whom we share a mutual obligation and with whom we walk in life. Like Humberto says, there is no *diferencia*. Yet, this distinction Humberto makes between we and them is based on cultural archetypes. If probed,

Humberto likely would agree that there are within-group differences and across-group similarities.

With *compañeros* we also find and re-create a home—the home we once had and from which we fled. It is the home that expelled us and the home we have been searching for since we left. This is what we find in getting involved, and it is one of the main reasons we stay involved. Home is where we belong, the space we can call ours, where we feel safe and protected; where we are not brown, Latinos, or Hispanics. Home is our shelter against the gendered and racialized world.

Humberto has been volunteering for several years at Shanti, in San Francisco. He approached the AIDS support organization after learning he was HIV positive. He relishes his time at Shanti. "I kind of see it as a job, because I go there Monday through Friday," he says. Volunteering at Shanti has provided him ample rewards. "Shanti has been real good to me. It has given me the ability to wake up in the morning and want to be there, all day if possible." Indeed, a few months before our conversation, he received an award for his volunteer work.

From the moment he joined Shanti, Humberto knew he had found a community of Latino gay men:

> I realized there were other Latinos there who were feeling some of the same feelings I was feeling. It was a place where I didn't have to feel impotent about what I felt. I was able to just say what I wanted without being made to feel less. I couldn't have said what I said then if it would have been in a white group.

The sense of home that he found among the *compañeros* allowed him to express himself without a fear of either being ignored or rejected. He developed self-confidence. This newfound power was a turning point. Until then, his life had been shattered by HIV:

> I learned a lot of things about HIV, about how others were feeling emotionally, physically, and spiritually. It just made it more OK—made me see I wasn't the only one. I got a lot of good friends out of that group.

Amid the community of HIV-positive people, Humberto grew in self-confidence. In joining the organization, he found others who were enduring the ravages of HIV and AIDS. He did not feel isolated, not the only one dealing with HIV and with the guilt and shame that it brings. Volunteering has helped him cope with HIV.

Through our community involvement, thus, we refurbish the stigma we have experienced because of our skin color, "unmanly" behavior, and AIDS. The stigma that we experienced up to this point in our lives had, for many of us, become part of our self-concept. We had come to see ourselves through the eyes of the oppressor, as a part of a lesser group. We had come to blame ourselves for our "shortcomings." We began to alter this view by joining a group and being among *compañeros*. We realized that our "shortcomings" are not of our own making. They do not even exist. They are the creation of the stigmatizer. There is nothing wrong with our skin color, with our accent, with our feminine manners, with our desire to love and to penetrate and be penetrated.

Humberto has also improved his self-image through his volunteer work with Shanti and other organizations:

> I'm hoping they can see I'm a good person. I'm a hard worker and I'm good at what I do. Everywhere I've volunteered, I've gotten a lot of acknowledgment for it and that's good for me. It makes me feel good. I'm not just trying to do something to make myself look good and then go on. I really want to do well and I really want to be remembered as doing good.

Volunteering and activism are intrinsically gratifying and feed our egos. We feel useful. In addition, by getting involved we find a purpose, which we are unable to find in other spheres. We find meaning in our lives, as has Humberto: "I just don't want to be a number, a statistic."

But there is something more that Humberto has learned through his volunteer work. He has acquired a new understanding of the people with whom he works and within his own community. He has discovered a sense of awareness about AIDS and its impact on people's lives:

> I think when I first got diagnosed I had this overwhelming thing of "I can barely take care of myself, how can I expect to help somebody else?" But going there [to Shanti], I learned a lot. I learned how to talk to the clients, be patient and listen to them. A lot of them are on the street. A lot of them are drug addicts, and a lot of them are homeless.
>
> I see clients on a daily basis. A lot of them come with the excuse of getting coupons, but they just wanted a couple of minutes to talk to somebody.
>
> It doesn't make me stronger, but it makes me more aware of what's going on around my community.

In this chapter I describe the changes brought about by community involvement. Community involvement works as an epiphany for these activists. It is a process whereby the "old self" is transformed into a new and different self (Denzin 1989; Hawkins 1990; Ramirez-Valles 1999).

Community activism produces long-term changes in one's life, bringing a new sense of self (McAdam 1989). Many successful changes usually follow a renegotiation of one's identity, giving rise to a new identity that is neither socially rejected nor stigmatized by others or oneself (Heatherton and Nichols 1994). The degree of change depends on the kind of activism and the "type of person we used to be."

Activists in social movements typically undergo two basic forms of personal change: conversion and, as we began to examine in chapter 5, alteration (McAdam 1989; Travisano 1981). Conversion entails a total disruption with the past. It implies a radical transformation of the self, social networks, and worldview and the adoption of an opposite and sometimes negated identity. Conversion tends to occur among groups with high cohesion and with strong opposition to mainstream society. On the other hand, we recall that alteration is a subtle change involving the same overall self-identity. It follows a pattern of development from existing ways of being and acting. Alteration is perceived as a "natural" change within the realm of one's identity and expectations; it takes place in less inclusive and in more open groups. This is the most common personal change I found among *compañeros*. Alteration is still a significant aspect of life as most people's changes come in this way.

The organizations these Latinos belong to, as well as the larger AIDS and gay movements, shape the personal changes activists undergo (Denzin 1989). The group provides them with information, a set of meanings, and a direction to change their lives. The group helps them to reinterpret old and new behaviors and to build an identity based on the group culture. The process of change is thus set up and made possible through the acquisition of a new set of meanings and acts. These newly gained elements are not individual. Rather, they are created and shared by *compañeros* in a group or organization.

Becoming a Latino Gay Man

This transformation created by community involvement yields two identities in one: Latino and gay. Though traditionally conflicted, they are elements of the same identity for many of these activists.

Luigi, who suffered cerebral palsy as a child, is thirty-six years old and volunteers with two Latino gay organizations in San Francisco. He says that when he came out as a gay person, he did not have any Latino peers. The Latinos were "kind of homophobic":

> All the other Hispanic guys I would see were attached to white guys, or they were very closeted and you just didn't want to look at them. *Como que te da pena, pobre gente* [You feel sorry for them, poor people].

Luigi explains that, after that experience, he "pushed aside" his Latino self:

> As a matter of fact, in the early '90s, I plunged in headfirst into the gay community, when I was first out, and I didn't see a lot of positive things as far as Latino men.

Through his work as a volunteer, Luigi had opportunities to meet other gay men from various Latin American countries, which in turn allowed him to speak in his first language, Spanish. This has enriched his life. He has a sense of belonging. "I do feel like I'm a part of the community." But most significantly, he was able to integrate his Latino self with his gay self:

> That actually changed my perception of being Latino, too. I think it's given me another identity. I'm a gay Latino in this city. I've worked for the Latino organizations and I'm openly gay as a volunteer. I'm part of a community, a gay Latino community. It's helped me because I view my sexuality as a Latino man. I don't separate it.
>
> It gives me an awareness that Latinos are a diverse community. Some of us are gay, some are openly gay. I've evolved. I am a completely different person. I know it's changed me.

Luigi has acquired a new sense of self as a Latino gay man. He attributes this to his participation as a volunteer in two Latino organizations for almost six years. In those organizations, he found a home, where he learned about other gay men, who eventually became his *compañeros*. His perceptions about Latino men being "macho" and "homophobic" changed.

The sense of community gives rise to the new sense of self. Pablo, a twenty-nine-year-old HIV-positive man, also volunteers in one of the organizations where Luigi volunteers. He explains that, prior to his involvement with the organization, he did not know where to find other Latinos. In the organization, he notes that guys can talk about being themselves away from the "oversexed" gay culture. Pablo has become acquainted with the diversity of Latinos who come from the Americas. Raised in a predominantly white neighborhood and schools, he felt disconnected from other Latinos. His volunteer work has helped restore his connection to the Latino culture and community in San Francisco:

> It's helped me immensely to open up to my own Latin culture. And now I feel like I'm part of it. I think that's the important part for me.

We must remember that the meaning of *Latino* is not settled. As a label and a group category in the racialized society of the United States, it is quite fractured. Some of us, especially immigrants, use the term reluctantly, while others use it with ease. In the context of activism and volunteerism, especially when it takes place among Latinos, the Latino identity takes precedence. The community and the *compañeros* we encounter exhort us to adopt a Latino identity, even if it is bounded by the community organization where we volunteer. It is the *convivencia* (coexistence) with *compañeros*, to borrow the words of one activist, George, which makes us look at ourselves as Latinos.

You might recall from previous chapters that Fabian identifies himself primarily as Mexican. As a relatively new immigrant to the United States, he thinks of himself as "Mexican, before Hispanic, before Latino." Shortly after arriving in Chicago, he adopted an identity as a gay man and got divorced. Then, he started volunteering for a group of Latino gay men. This experience has led him to see himself as a Latino (or Hispanic). He says:

> Yet because I got involved with the Hispanic gay group, I feel more Hispanic. I have more years in the United States, but I begin to feel part of a Hispanic group . . . it feels nice to find people like myself. I feel part of a group. I also feel part of this country, which before I didn't. Now I feel more American and Hispanic, and Latino.

For Fabian, as for many of us, the sense of community and belonging is what adopting the Latino identity means. We find it when we join others in a organization or movement. The *compañeros* we make and the identity we adopt also help us find our place in the world, specifically in a racialized society. Fabian explains:

> I feel more integrated. I feel a part of Chicago and the United States. That is, a part of U.S. society, because I begin to see myself as a part of an ethnic group, of a community. I have come a long way in the four years since I came out of the closet.

Fabian now feels at ease as a Latino and a gay man. These two aspects of his new identity (albeit not completely settled), did not exist for him when living in Mexico as a professional, middle-class married man. His community involvement has been a crucial element in that transition.

Along with the newly acquired identity as a Latino gay man comes a strengthened self-image, or, as Eliezer calls it, a feeling of empowerment:

> [My volunteer work] has fortified my self-esteem. I feel more secure as a person. For example, when I participated in the Queers of Color event, it was a step forward for me. I was presenting myself not as a gay man, but as a Latino gay man.
> Perhaps because of my fair skin color, many people would think I was white. But when I presented myself as a queer of color, I was including myself as a Latino. It has been a way to empower myself and the way I think of myself.

An activist from California, Armando has undergone a parallel transformation. When he was younger, he was unhappy about being brown, gay,

and poor. In high school he became goth. Then, his life began to change
after finishing college in the Northeast:

> I felt like the volunteer work solidified for me what it is to be gay and Latino.
> Like it's OK to be both. And there're all these people here that are like me. At
> college, I never had gay Latino friends. I never even had gay friends. Then when
> I came out here, I suddenly have all these gay Latino friends, who I have a lot
> of things in common with.
>
> That's what empowerment is. It's communicating, sharing, and connecting
> with people who have had similar stuff as you.

As we might expect, not everybody in this group speaks of this type of
transformation. The saliency of this identity change and of Latino and gay
identities varies as well. For a minority of these activists, like Eric, community involvement altered only their identities as gay men. Eric, a forty-six-
year-old Puerto Rican, first volunteered for the Metropolitan Community
Church. Later, when he became involved with a group of Latino gay men
in Chicago, he came to see himself as a gay man:

> One time, I decided to visit the church and it was wonderful. I became a delegate
> of the church. I met a lot of friends. And then the [Latino group] came. I started
> with the organization and got involved with meetings and with forums. That's
> how I got all my friends. It did change me. That's how I was able to accept my-
> self. I was able to meet friends and was able to contribute to other gay Latinos.

For an exceptional few of the activists, community involvement had little
impact on their identities. Eduardo is one activist who claims volunteering
in the AIDS movement did not change his image as either a gay or a Latino
man:

> I had a boyfriend. I'd go to gay bars. I wasn't out with my family. I wasn't
> out to anybody at work. I wanted to be more out. That's why I joined the gay
> group. It made me feel like I was actually a little bit more out, but it didn't
> make me more active. I wasn't an activist. I'm glad I volunteered, but in terms
> of fundamental changes, no.

After leaving Texas, Eduardo was living what we would call a gay life in
California. He had live-in boyfriends, gay friends, and he was socializing
with other gay men when he volunteered for the AIDS Walk. His family
was not fully aware of his life as a gay man, however. He became involved
with a gay group, in addition to volunteering for the AIDS Walk. Although
he found some *compañeros* and a sense of belonging, his views of himself
as a Latino gay man did not change. Nor did the way in which he related
with his family change.

Development of the Gay and Transgender Self

While community involvement might not always transform the way we see ourselves in relation to an ethnic group or a gender system, it can alter our identities by deepening them or by accentuating less stigmatized aspects of those identities.

Alexis speaks of this change in terms of getting a "sense of normality." He explains that through his involvement he has learned about himself and others. "It opened up my eyes." Being involved, he says, has made him feel that "It's OK to be gay." He has discovered that what he had experienced and felt is quite common; there are others with whom he shares a similar path. Alexis has found role models among the *compañeros* and has become a stronger person. He feels "normal": "I feel as if I were heterosexual."

An immigrant from El Salvador, Mario always wanted to dress up and perform as a woman. His concerns about the stigma of cross-dressing stopped him from ever trying it. Now, at the age of fifty, and thanks partly to his involvement in a group of Latino gay men in San Francisco, he is able to realize his dream:

> I was always an artist, but as a man; as a man dressed as a man. Now I have had the strength to perform on stage dressed as a woman. I love it. I love it because that's who I am. I'm not ashamed of whatever my family would say. I'm doing what I want to do.

In this type of change produced by community involvement, the basic concept of the self does not change. What changes is the manner in which we see ourselves as either Latino or GBT. Activists and volunteers such as Alexis and Mario can overcome the stigma they have experienced and internalized and express themselves. They now have a wider spectrum of choices to be who they are and want to be.

Bernardo offers another example of this type of change. He has been successful in his professional career, but he cannot fully express himself as most nongay colleagues can, in his workplace. He accepts the fact that he can not be an openly gay man at work. "I think it is OK for what it is. I can't force it out of them, but it's just a very straight environment." However, he has found a space to be himself as a gay and Latino man in his volunteer work:

> So when I go to meetings at the organization, I see my friends and we kiss on the lips. I don't necessarily act any different than I do at work, but it's kind of like when you go back home, to Mexico. You speak in your own language and you talk about friends and family. It's just a different world all of a sudden. So that's why I feel like I have a gay community.

The people on the front lines of AIDS are fighting HIV and AIDS, but they are also changing themselves and the *compañeros* around them. Paradoxically, in the process of affirming themselves as GBT, some of them unintentionally re-create images of the "good" and the "bad" GBT. Victor's story illustrates this process. He became active in AIDS and LGBT issues through his partner. Victor explains that his involvement has helped him accept himself and find a community:

> It makes me like more accepting towards myself, and more identified with the community . . . being more accepting in being known as being gay.

But through his involvement, Victor has also discovered the "good," or positive, as well as the not-so-good aspects of such a community:

> It also helps me see that it's not only that stereotypical community, the promiscuous community, just out to have fun. It's also that we want our rights and we deserve our rights. It does allow me to see that there is promiscuity in it, but that there's also a good side of it. We're not all about going out and having fun. We also want a regular life and kids. We want the right to live with our partners.

The image that Victor has created through his volunteer work is also good for his family. He explains:

> My mom is happy, because she was scared of the stereotype. She's happy that I'm not into that and that we're actually fighting for our rights.

Victor is emphasizing that his family is perhaps accepting of his sexuality and his live-in partner because they are not only about "having fun" and "promiscuity." Thus, in an effort to create a normalized image of themselves for their own use and for others to see, some *compañeros* reproduce the stigma toward GBT. In other words, as they rework the stigma they have experienced and internalized to create a positive self, they endorse some of society's negative attitudes toward those who do not conform to the dominant gender roles and sexual mores of the general society.

Ignacio, who has been volunteering since his teenage years, speaks in similar terms about his image as a gay man and his mother's views:

> I try to expose [my parents] as much as I can. I'd go home and I'd talk about like, "Oh, you know, we're having a gay pride parade." My mom is like: "Oh, *para qué* [what for]?" But now she understands that in high school I was an activist. I did things to make the LGBT committee visible.
>
> I told her—'cause she has this image that I'm really going out to clubs and screwing men, and I'm going to be all scandalous, doing drugs and stuff—"No, you didn't raise me like that. I know better and I'm glad that you raised me how I am."

Community involvement helps us create an identity that is less stigmatized. But it might also be a way for us to compensate for the negative aspects of the self, whether gay, transgender, or an HIV-positive self.

Development of the HIV-positive and Sexual Self

Two other aspects of the self are altered through community involvement: the identity as a stigmatized HIV-positive person and the manner in which the self deals with the risk of HIV.

Heriberto is thirty-eight years old and lives in San Francisco. He came to the United States from Brazil in search of HIV treatments. He joined an AIDS organization because he wanted to learn more about his new status as a person living with HIV. Through the organization he realized that he was not the only one struggling with HIV, and he found support:

> At one time, the group was like my life. I used to spend my days there. It was like my family. It was my first volunteer work ever. I felt very proud of me to be able to help other people. And I made good friends and I learned so much. I felt I was doing something good for somebody.

Over his years of volunteering, Heriberto has made many friends. Some of them have already died of AIDS-related causes. As Heriberto says, helping others nourishes the self, enabling one to feel useful and gratified. It also provides a point of comparison with *compañeros*. We compare our own selves and experiences with those of *compañeros* and others that we help, as they walk similar paths and are living under similar circumstances.

In Chicago, Guillermo, also living with HIV, attests to this effect of helping others:

> Volunteering had made it a lot easier for me to deal with my own HIV. It's made it so much easier to deal with it in helping other people. When I think I've got some big issues, personally, at home, relationships, housing, a tremendous gas bill, or when I think about what am I going to do with my life, I get a chance to witness first hand other people's issues. Sometimes they have to deal with them all alone. Then I realize my problems aren't that bad and . . . sounds cliché-ish, but you walk out of here being very thankful that you just are not in their shoes.

When the point of comparison is not the Other (e.g., the HIV-negative or the heterosexual man), but *compañeros,* those with whom we share common experiences, our self-image changes in a positive way.

Marc, another activist living with HIV, reaffirms that sentiment when he says, "I feel good when I help others." But Marc, who grew up in Peru, also speaks of an outcome of joining that we have seen before: the ability to shield society's stigma toward those living with HIV and AIDS. He explains:

> It has given me the courage and the strength not to get down because of what others say about me. "Well, I'm positive; I don't care what people say." I have learned to value and accept myself as a positive person. I don't fear people talking bad about me. Before, I was scared.

The company of others who are like us—in this instance, those who live with HIV—helps us to see ourselves through our own eyes, which are also the eyes of our *compañeros*. This is one way in which joining alters stigmatized identities.

In the time of AIDS, it is not easy to have sex. It is not easy to be a gay man or a transgender person and enjoy the pleasures of the flesh. The medical and public health discourse has taken over our sex lives as well. Now, many of us have to negotiate the mandates of the HIV-risk discourse with those of the heart and the flesh. Involvement, especially in AIDS organizations, gives us a place to speak about our fear of HIV, our uncertainties about safe sex, our displeasure for condoms, and our ways of overcoming those fears and doubts.

In my interviews with these activists, we talked about sex, specifically about having sex with other men. The topic elicited a variety of reactions and conversational tones. While most were open, frank, and even witty when talking about their sexual behaviors, other activists were reserved, and still a few evaded the matter completely. Yet we almost always found a consensus on the difficulty of practicing safe sex. The use of condoms is not universally consistent among these activists or for each individual. Many agree, however, that involvement has helped address the need to use condoms and the nuisance of safe sex.

I asked Carmelo: "What did you learn from all the work you have done?" He answered: "It made my sex life safer. I mean, it's always condoms. Sometimes it's without condoms, but nobody's screwing anybody." I probed further and asked him: "So, if no condoms, nobody's screwing?" "Right," he answered. He then explains:

> In my case, I'm always careful when I'm about to have sex with somebody; I always check them up physically. Besides AIDS, there's other stuff you can catch, like crabs. So I learned to do that. I think because I have talked about other stuff with people, I don't get as nervous talking about sex and what I've learned, I've been involved in teaching.

Carmelo is part of the cohort of gay men who was hit the hardest by the epidemic. He was in his early thirties when HIV emerged. He lost his partner of that time to AIDS, but he is HIV negative. He has also been active in the AIDS movement since the early years of the epidemic. He has volunteered in several AIDS and LGBT organizations, including conducting basic education about HIV and AIDS in high schools and colleges. Those experiences have made it easier for him to incorporate safe sex into his life as a gay man.

Some of the activists who are living with HIV also reflect on the changes that their involvement has produced in their sexual practices. One of them, Jimmy, explains that even before volunteering, he knew about HIV and safe-sex protocols. But he did not apply what he knew. "Right now, I couldn't have sex with someone without a condom. I have learned a lot." He credits this change to his participation in a Chicago-area AIDS organization. Jimmy's guiding principle is "I don't want to do as they did to me."

Development of the Self

Other changes created through community involvement are not directly related to the self-identity, but do contribute to the development of the self. This includes acquiring self-confidence, professional skills, self-esteem, and the understanding of others.

Isidro was twenty-years old when he joined ACT UP in San Francisco. There, he found his first role model, a Latino gay man who was one of the leaders of the organization. In this leader, he saw the possibility of being both a Latino and a gay man:

> He was a brown face amongst the sea of white faces in leather jackets. He was fiercely Latino and fiercely queer. That was just like, "Wow! There is another option for me."

Isidro was among the youngest in the organization, but the inspiration he had from seeing the Latino leader pushed him to take leadership roles as well:

> I was certainly the youngest on the board at the time. I just sort of walked in and—don't take no prisoners—I spoke my mind. I think that's what ACT UP helped me do. Actually, growing up, I was always quiet and not really one to voice my opinion. Even in college, they would throw a dig at me for a response. Then being part of ACT UP just sort of taught me to assert myself.

That same sense of newfound assertiveness is echoed by Jack, who identifies himself as the "HIV-positive poster child." After leaving the AIDS organization where he started volunteering, Jack went on to form a new organization in the Midwest:

> [My activism] made me believe. I was learning along the way, because I never ran an organization. I was a factory worker. It made me believe I could move

mountains if I wanted to. It made me believe that God was very [present] in all of it. It changed me.

Isidro and Jack served in leadership roles and remained visible figures in their own contexts. They undertook major responsibilities in their respective organizations. Thus, upon learning their stories, we can appreciate the drastic changes that they underwent. Even small-scale tasks or actions can positively impact our sense of confidence. Ismael, for example, says that he became so sure of himself as a result of his involvement in his company's LGBT group that he marched in the Gay Pride Parade. "I marched with my huge banner. It was [my partner's and my] first time. I felt very good doing it."

This sense of confidence sometimes comes with learning new skills, expanding one's horizons as an activist or as a professional. These days, Gregorio is well-known in Chicago for his leadership, especially among HIV-positive people. He coordinates a support program for HIV-positive Latino men and has been on the Prevention Planning Council for several years. He regularly participates as a reviewer for HIV- and AIDS-related grant proposals in the local health department and in the Centers for Disease Control and Prevention (CDC).

But it took several years for Gregorio to get to this point. It all began when he was diagnosed with HIV. He then joined a support group, part of the program he now coordinates. He explains that the guys in the group forced him to learn and get involved with other groups, as they would ask him questions about new medications and services available for people living with HIV and AIDS. "They were the ones who pushed me to learn more," he says.

Gregorio got involved in several national advocacy groups. "I began to apply for money to participate in conferences, because I wanted to learn so much. I have been very fortunate that I have always gotten the funds." He tells the story of his first visit to Washington, D.C., where he discovered a new identity:

> I was invited to speak in a panel on prevention for people living with HIV. They introduced me as an activist living with AIDS. I almost cried. I was never referred to as an activist.

Gregorio's long-term involvement has changed his life in many ways, but most significantly it has changed his self-confidence. He has been pushed by his *compañeros* and by himself to seek out new territories. He has become a self-assured AIDS activist at the national level.

For these activists, newly acquired knowledge, new social relations, and their work in their communities provide them with skills and abilities they can apply to themselves and in their relationships with others. For them, community involvement does not transform their basic sense of themselves. Rather, it helps in their development of the self.

In the preceding stories, we already glimpsed a connection between self-confidence and self-esteem. As our self-confidence increases and we redefine the experienced and internalized stigma through joining, our self-image also improves. Ramón, who is fifty-one years old and HIV positive, says: "I love my work. I feel useful. It gives me a lot of strength to go on."

Ramón became involved in 1991, a year after he tested positive. His community work has become a necessity. "It's like a part of my daily life." Over the years, he has accumulated five awards in recognition of his activism. His activism has changed his self-image. "It has changed me from the point of view that I feel very good about myself."

Jimmy, also an activist living with HIV, explains:

> I enjoy it [activism]. When I see that I accomplish something, it makes me happy, I feel useful knowing that I'm contributing something. It makes me feel good to connect with other people. It has made me more human, more centered, and less selfish.

In simple and direct language, Bernardo says of his volunteer work on the board of an AIDS organization: "I guess I do get off of being on the board."

One of the areas in which Renato is trying to make a difference is in access to HIV drugs. As I noted in chapter 6, from San Francisco he started an AIDS drug-recycling program to Cuba. He helps collect medicines in the United States and sends them to Cuba, where a small organization distributes them free of charge. Through this activism he has become conscious of the circumstances of other people's lives:

> It made me aware of the suffering and poverty that I've never seen. It made me not take for granted a lot of things.
>
> When I went to Cuba, I got extremely affected by my experience. The level of hunger is such that you would even behave on a sexual orientation that is different from yours, if that would bring you money and food. But seeing twelve-year-olds prostituting themselves for American males, or a Canadian man, or Spanish men. . . . Right there on the street I saw firsthand a persecution of gay men from the police.

This is the critical consciousness that activism may also create in us. Through our involvement in the world, we learn about others' perspectives and realities. We realize that there are other ways of experiencing the world and come to see ourselves as agents, as active members of the world. And we acquire what Paolo Freire (1971) calls a critical consciousness. That is, we see the inherent contradictions of social class, race, or a gender-based system, and the possibilities for change.

In the next excerpt, Gonzalo describes his experience working in the Bronx. Through the details of his story, we see the critical consciousness created through involvement. Gonzalo moved from the West Coast to New York City as part of a church program. It was in the early years of the epidemic, and he ended up working in an underground needle-exchange program and with sex workers, led by a priest. As did Renato, he came to understand the wider social context of the HIV epidemic:

> The neighborhood was not exactly the prettiest. I had never done this before and I felt that I was going against everything that I was supposed to stand for.
>
> It was really exciting. I was doing it gladly in a sense, because I knew that after four weeks it was going to be over. It was getting depressing . . . seeing the condition of these human beings, seeing how they're treated and seeing that they're out there to make a buck on top of all of this. They have to go through abuse and the risk of having a customer come and give them some disease or something.
>
> The stories they would tell us. . . . They were blamed. . . . They were spat on. They were hit. The weather and the scene was not helping either. It's not like we were in a beautiful park. There were train tracks everywhere, and cars that were dismantled everywhere. The houses were falling apart. It was snowing. It was cold.

At the time, Gonzalo was in his early twenties. The experience shaped his views on the epidemic and on those marginalized groups. "It made me see the seriousness of the disease and its ramifications. It also helped me see sex workers as human beings."

In these preceding stories, the transformative power of community involvement is clearer than before. The identity is not altered. Rather, the way in which we act in the world and how we relate with others changes. We develop a strong sense of ourselves, as Latino and GBT. We also obtain a critical consciousness. We see ourselves as actors, as opposed to passive subjects in the world, and we see the world as sustaining and reproducing systems of inequality based on social class, race, and gender.

Actualization of the Self

Mateo first got involved in Mexico, before he emigrated to the United States. As a teenager he participated in the Catholic youth movement and later did outreach with an AIDS organization. On a personal level, he derived a great sense of satisfaction trying to affect some change in the AIDS epidemic.

His satisfaction comes from contributing with his "granito de arena" (little grain of sand):

> In Mexico many people have taboos, stigma, and are hypocritical, partly due to the religion. Many were fearful of HIV and AIDS. That was the point of our labor, to raise people's awareness. We wanted people to understand and learn about HIV to protect themselves by using condoms, especially in the gay community.
>
> It is a personal satisfaction to help others. You feel proud of doing that. You feel good about yourself.

An activist from Brazil, Ramiro says, "I think I have gotten more than I have given." Like Mateo, he feels great satisfaction from working for others:

> Until this day people approach me and say, "You have saved my life," "you have changed my life." I have gotten this immense gratification as a human being. . . . What is cooler than to be doing prevention work around AIDS being a gay man?

This chapter concludes with one last, yet important change brought about through joining: the actualization of the self. Unlike previously discussed changes, this type of change does not alter the self; it only allows the self to be and to unfold. Here, volunteering and activism provide the space to express the self and obtain satisfaction and recognition.

Satisfaction and recognition, as described by Mateo and Ramiro, are part of a relevant concept in the actualization of the self through community involvement: "mattering," which means that we know we are important to others and that we are valuable parts of a group or community (Elliot et al. 2004). It means that others acknowledge our contributions to the group and to the community (Schieman and Taylor 2001). As the stories of Mateo and Ramiro illustrate, mattering is tied to our self-esteem. We feel good about ourselves because we know we are important in the lives of others, our *compañeros*.

Pierre, who is pursuing graduate religious studies, says this of mattering: "It is a satisfaction, better than preaching a sermon in church. Preaching is not as effective in contributing." George also links mattering to self-image:

> I feel good about myself and I know I'm doing something for others. It's something you have deep inside you. If we all put our *granito de arena* [little grain of sand] in our community, it could get better.

For some of these activists, especially those who are highly involved and hold leadership positions, recognition is one of the most important results of their involvement. They want to make a difference in others' lives, but they also want to be recognized for doing that. They relish the leadership that they have gained through their hard, unpaid, work.

I had known Gerardo for a few years before we did the interview for this study. I saw him as a leader not only in the Latino LGBT community, but also in the larger Latino and gay LGBT communities. That's how I met him. Others repeatedly told me about him and his work. But it was not until our interview that I learned how hard he has worked on behalf of Latinos (hence, his position as a leader) and how much he cared about our recognition and respect. He says:

> It makes me a player. I know that people worry about my opinion. What makes me feel good is people know to come to me. People know I can be helpful. Some of them may not like me, some of them might think: "He's always got his own opinion and agenda." People know that I'm connected.
>
> So, that's one of things my community involvement sort of brought me. I know that when people say, "Oh, is there a Latino leader?" And especially if they add the other adjective, a *gay* Latino leader, I'm going to be in the list. It's nice to know that I've made my mark.

Gregorio, who I also have known for about eight years in Chicago, says he likes getting the recognition for his work with youths and HIV-positive Latinos. "I like being recognized and being told that I'm giving a lot to the people I work for in the community." He is not shy about his enjoyment of acknowledgment and honor. "I'm fascinated by diplomas and awards."

This idea of mattering, as seen in Gerardo and Gregorio's excerpts, may sound somewhat egotistical. I believe there is a part of mattering that is self-centered. Some of us might not embrace it because we, as either volunteers or activists, follow the morally accepted script that we do the work without expecting any reward or recognition. Yet, the difference here is that mattering is an outcome of a task deeply appreciated, making a difference with *compañeros*.

This is made clearer in Hernan's account. He explains that he has developed leadership skills through his involvement in Aguilas in San Francisco. "Cultivating leadership and influencing people." He enjoys having a say in the organization and having an impact on others' lives. He adds that part of his role is to foster leadership by offering "a place where people can get started and connected with others, and develop in whatever direction they want to go in." Notably, the satisfaction and recognition that he gets are the product of working with others:

> A lot of us who do this get satisfaction out of creating an event or a safe environment for people to come and be themselves. Be it Latino, be it gay. But at the same time, there are social and political issues that need to be addressed and so that was the other part of this group that evolved.

We should not allow these stories about change to lead us to romanticize community involvement. Community involvement may create burnout and conflict (the latter is not always a negative aspect of a movement or organization). I experienced both during my work in the Mexico–United States border region. In the AIDS organization we were part of in Ciudad Juárez, Oscar, Marco, and I had an intense argument over the management of some funds, which hurt our friendship (we repaired the damage years later). One of the reasons I left the border and my work with my *compañeros* to go to Michigan was burnout. I had lost some of the excitement and felt unchallenged.

I have witnessed burnout and conflict among other *compañeros* in the United States. And we have seen glimpses of them in the stories in this book, though we did not explore these issues in depth during the interviews with the activists. Yet, many of the activists with whom I talked have stopped their community involvement at some point in their lives, due to burnout and conflicts they faced within the organizations. Other activists have moved from one organization to another because they have had differences or clashes with members, staff, or leaders.

The changes that community involvement fosters are real and significant. Yet again, the conclusion is not a cheerful outlook on life, which these changes seem to portray. The lives of these activists, as Latinos, gay, and transgender persons, do not end when they become volunteers or activists. The struggles of the *compañeros,* their families, and their societies, persist. Some of them made this point clear to me when I shared with them some of my conclusions from the interviews. They agreed, for the most part, with my interpretation of the data. But they told me the ending looked "too rosy." They are right. Certainly, AIDS is still an epidemic. The racial, class, and gender system that organizes our lives has not weakened, and in fact it has perhaps strengthened. And in our personal lives we continue to face new challenges.

THE ROAD OF COMPAÑEROS

We had driven for two hours, when Marco asked me to stop and turn back. We were on our way to Chihuahua, the state's capital, to meet with a group of gay men who were working on HIV and AIDS. A *compañera* we met in the women's health organization for which I was working in Ciudad Juárez had put us in contact with the group. Older than us and a product of the student movement of the late 1960s in Mexico, Patsy was a hippie. She lived in Chihuahua and knew of this small group of men who had come together to fight HIV and AIDS, but had no financial resources. Patsy thought we could provide some guidance. I borrowed my brother's pickup truck, and Marco and I were driving there for a long weekend.

But Marco was not feeling well. At first I attributed his mood to one of his not-so-rare impulsive and stubborn outbursts. He was afraid and anxious. The week before, we had taken our first HIV tests. José drew the blood from us in his house and sent it to the lab, via the clinic where he was employed. I had forgotten about it already, but Marco hadn't. On the road, he asked me to return to Juárez. He thought his result would come back positive. He was pretty sure. He wanted to be alone on the second floor of his parents' house in the bedroom he had claimed as his own. I made a half-hearted attempt to change his mind, having always respected his opinions and his own peculiar way of being, while he always respected mine.

I started to turn the truck around, but Marco stopped me. "Never mind," he said. "Forget about me; let's keep going."

I got a little angry but continued driving to Chihuahua. Marco had changed his mind because of the commitment we had made with the guys in Chihuahua. That commitment was more important than our individual worries and troubles. As it turns out, we had a fantastic time in Chihuahua.

We met with the guys and visited a couple of gay bars. And our test results came back negative.

Months later, we were in El Paso's airport. I was leaving for Michigan to begin graduate school, and Marco had come to say good-bye. I had missed my flight because the lines to cross the border between Ciudad Juárez and El Paso were too long and moving very slowly (we on the border think the gringos and the immigration officers want to make the crossing as inconvenient as possible). So, we had plenty of time to kill as I waited for the next flight. Marco stayed with me the several hours before my departure. My plans were to return to Mexico after finishing my master's degree. I might not go to Juárez—perhaps to Mexico City. In any event, I would go somewhere in Mexico. Marco suspected otherwise. He told me I was not coming back.

He was right: I have been in United States since then, visiting Mexico and Juárez only occasionally.

Compañeros are at the heart of this book. I discovered *compañeros* while working on this book, reading through thousands of pages of transcripts, cutting and pasting excerpts, and translating words and passages. I did not start this research with the idea of *compañeros,* or with a question about *compañeros.* I found them along the road and after a couple of years working on this project. They probably have been there all along. I just did not see them before. I realized that *compañeros* are an essential quality of our volunteerism and activism as Latino GBTs. They constitute a force that drives us to come together. They are the glue that keeps us together.

But we should avoid essentialism. Being a *compañero* is not in our skin color, in our Spanish language, or in our accented and broken English language. It is not a quality inherent in being Latino, a gay man, or a transgender person. In the same manner that Latino is not a natural quality or a quality based on skin color, neither is *compañeros.* It is not the way all Latinos relate; it is not a universal relationship among Latino GBTs. *Compañerismo* is a quality of a type of relationship created through participation in a social-movement organization or a small group that has come together, explicitly or implicitly, for a common cause and against an amorphous yet real enemy. It is a quality that emerges from ties of solidarity among the socially marginalized. It is created in a cultural context, such as the Humboldt Park neighborhood in Chicago, the Mission District in San Francisco, or Santiago de Chile, where interpersonal bonds and cooperation come before individualism, private life, and competition. This form of relating to others is a cultural code—hence, difficult to decipher to the outsider.

In this form of relationship and coexistence rests the possibility for resistance and creative power. *Compañeros,* as a concept, is more than a source of support and comfort; it can also be a creative force through which we resist assimilation, accommodation, racism, and homophobia. It also enables us to forge alternative ways of being. This form of being with others, unlike marriage, has the potential to provide an alternative space for us to be. It can even change how the heterosexual world relates.

Twenty-five years after the first AIDS case was diagnosed, the social movement it produced is now stagnant. The radical agenda and approach that once characterized the AIDS movement are tamed, if not gone. Also gone are the anger, the creative energy, and the vibrant solidarity. The same can be said about the gay movement. In the 1980s, the gay and the AIDS movements became one; now, the former has separated. It has minimized AIDS, embraced a conservative agenda, and pushed for assimilation into a heterosexual (and white) world.

This sentiment is shared by some queer voices in the United States (Crimp 2002; Harris 1997). In a recent interview, the film director Arthur Dong was asked about the state of gay and queer people in the United States:

> I'm disappointed, and at the same time, I'm elated at the progress that's been made. There is so much progress, and so much cause of celebration. At the same time, I think we are still very naïve. We're just not questioning the status quo. I don't know why our community doesn't do that. We're not fighting back. We're no getting ugly anymore. We're making everything pretty and acceptable. I lament the [passing of the] days of the Gay Liberation Front and ACT UP, I'll tell you. (Quoted in Varner 2005, 30–31)

The state of the AIDS and gay movements is partly due to their success. Funding for HIV and AIDS research and prevention has increased for many years. We have some access, albeit limited, to the research and funding agenda of federal and state agencies. Although treatments for HIV have been relatively successful in the United States, access is still a major concern. While AIDS and LGBT nonprofit organizations have sprouted up across the country, many of them were created by and for the white gay sector of the population.

Yet the fate of those movements has been shaped by other related factors. Perhaps the most important element is that the epidemic has turned black and brown. While HIV treatments have become widely available and successful among the majority of the white population, HIV infection continues to grow among African American and Latino people (CDC 2006). Moreover, among these groups, HIV detection is usually late and the success of HIV treatments is limited. Thus, for many white gay men, AIDS has lost its sense of appeal and urgency. What remains appealing to many white (and middle-class) gay men are the volunteering and fund-raising aspects of AIDS. They are interested in helping the Other, the "disenfranchised," and the AIDS patient. They are interested in putting on a tuxedo to attend galas and fashion shows.

The proliferation of nonprofit organizations delivering AIDS and LGBT-related services has gradually contained the movement. Many of these organizations were established as an arm of the state health agencies. They received funding to provide basic health services and collect data, as dictated by the National Institutes of Health and the Centers for Disease Control and Prevention. As the number of organizations grew, competition (as opposed to collaboration) became a part of the AIDS movement. The organizations led by African American and Latinos were frequently the victims, struggling to compete for funding with the white-controlled organizations. Money became the priority, sacrificing creativity and solidarity. The creative energy that many of us saw in the late 1980s and 1990s was channeled into writing grant proposals and filling out paperwork.

Moreover, many of us grew tired, while others became fearful of sex (Crimp 2002). Many gay men went the easy route and took refuge in the ideas of monogamy and safe sex. They drew a line between themselves and those who dared to continue being different by challenging the social and scientific discourses. Hoping to leave AIDS behind in part because of the fact that they saw AIDS as a by-product of the gay and sexual liberation movements, they embraced assimilation into the heterosexual white middle class. Now, many gay men do not want to be different from the heterosexual white middle class. They want to imitate it, including its hypocritical outlook. They want to get married, raise children, go to church, drive an SUV, and have a house in a nice neighborhood. At the same time, they want the freedom to have as many sexual partners as they wish.

There is nothing radical in marriage (Franke 2006; Josephson 2005). Indeed, marriage is a retrograde institution. It is one of the pillars of stigmatization for LGBT people; it gives rise to homophobia. I do welcome the fight for equality, but not the means. I agree that everyone should have access to benefits now assigned to those legally married, but why do I have to marry to have access to those benefits? Would having access to marriage and its benefits erase stigmatization and the accompanying discrimination for the LGBT population and people of color? No. Would it lessen social-class differences? No.

There are signs of the current state of the AIDS and gay movements in the life stories of these *compañeros*. There is not a collective agenda or ideology that guides their community involvement. What seems to guide their activism is a set of not-so-coherent issues, which very much reflect the political culture of the United States. The political environment of the United States is not about competing ideologies but issues. Potentially competing ideologies were eliminated in the 1960s. In the United States, the basic ideological system, the dominant set of values, call it capitalism or liberal democracy, is not questioned anymore. The political fights are about rights and issues, such as same-sex marriage and the so popular and frequently empty "isms": racism and sexism.

Only a minority of these Latino activists articulate an ideological agenda. They speak of social class and question the principles of liberal democracy and the hegemonic presence of the United States abroad. HIV, AIDS, and sexuality are embedded in the larger concepts of social class, capitalism, and democracy. But this is a minority. They developed their political and activist framework through college education and contact with particular leaders or role modes. AIDS and LGBT organizations, except for ACT UP, had little influence in the formation of their agenda.

Still, the potential for social change rests in relations of solidarity and obligation, like *compañerismo*. This, I argue, is one of those alternative forms of being and relating that Foucault talked about in the later part of his life. Speaking against the sexualization of homosexuality, he invites us to explore and develop alternative relationships that could provide the space to reinvent ourselves as gay, lesbian, or transgender beings, and break away from the norms of religion, family, and political structures (Eribon 2004).

Of course, I do not think Foucault was ever exposed to the experience or the concept of *compañeros*. He developed his ideas about new modes of relation among homosexual men from his own activism in France and his (limited) exposure to gay life in the United States, especially the leather gay subculture in the Bay Area. I have no experience to comment on the types of relationships evolving from the so-called leather scene, but I doubt we could find the type of relationship we are talking about here in the broader, mostly white, gay culture, perhaps with the exception of the ACT UP of the 1980s-1990s. The individualism is deeply rooted in the overall life plan and the everyday life of (white) individuals that makes it difficult to create relationships of solidarity and obligation among equals. Yet that is what makes *compañerismo* potentially subversive in the United States.

The potential to reinvent ourselves as Latino and LGBT people does not rest on our sexual acts, on our sexuality, or in marriage. It is in our ability to create and sustain alternative ways of being, which not only free us from social norms but allow us to contest power in whatever form it might take, either as an epidemic, or religious and economic values. Of this potential, Foucault noted, "not only do we have to defend ourselves, but also affirm ourselves, and affirm ourselves not only as an identity but as a creative force" (quoted in Eribon 2004: 323).

Is it possible to expand bonds of obligation and solidarity across ethnic groups? Can we have black and white *compañeros*? Yes, we can, and I think we currently do, but these are not easy tasks. Aside from the practical, yet important, elements of language differences and racial geographic segregation (after all, we usually do not live in the same neighborhoods), we have two other challenging factors. One is the current racial system. Our white peers must join us in the fight against it. The other is the ingrained individualism, particularly among our white peers. The normative individualism prevents them from feeling obligated to others, from giving themselves to others, and from being with others in communion. Individualism runs against building ties of solidarity and creating collective spaces, in the physical and spiritual sense. White gay men, thus, must get closer to others, instead of constantly maintaining a cool distance. They must open up their homes and souls. And they must not be afraid of being vulnerable.

A few days ago, I received an email from one of my nephews. After apologizing for not writing in several months, he asked for help. He needed to talk to me as soon as possible. He also asked me to keep it "between us." As I read and reread the email in an attempt to guess what was behind those words, memories ran through my mind of my conversations with him, of the time he visited me, and of the times I babysat him. And of course, the feeling I have always had recurred: he is gay.

The last conversation we had (before this latest email, also over email) was about *Brokeback Mountain*. After seeing the movie, he emailed me that he had thought of me and that it was "the best movie" he had ever seen (he is only twenty-two years old, so I excused him). Over several emails, he glorified the movie (unlike me) and the two male characters who fall in love but cannot be together. He also told me that El Paso, where he lives, still has a small-town culture. Gay people are not respected; they are mistreated. He also told me that he has several gay friends and frequently speaks out in their defense. In one of my replies, I told him, "Now you know why I left."

My feeling that he is gay and that he was using the movie to tell me. That was corroborated by every email we exchanged after that. Why would he tell me about the movie otherwise? I began writing to him, assuming that he is gay and was struggling because the people around him are not supportive. I shared with him a little of my own coming-out process. When I was about eighteen years old, I saw the movie *Making Love* on television. It is about a married man who goes out cruising one night through what seemed like a gay cruising or prostitution area. He picks up a handsome man and they fall in love. I thought it was a great movie. My reaction to that movie was similar to my nephew's response to *Brokeback Mountain*. The next day, I told my friend Maria Luisa about it. At that time, I did not know I was gay, but Maria Luisa deduced I was, though she did not say anything. Years later, we would laugh about it.

My nephew had said he would check out the movie. Then, in what would be the last email of that conversation, he wrote that he went to see the movie with "this girl that I'm seeing."

This time, his call for help, besides resuscitating my feelings about his sexual orientation, worries me. I ask for a phone number (because he changes his mobile phone number quite frequently) and the best time to call him. I return home late that evening and check my email. There is his reply. Anxiously, I open the email and my feeling is confirmed:

> I know that you are gay and, well, so am I. But I'm having a huge problem with it. You know how my parents are. They kinda know and they already told me that they would never accept me. I'm going through hell with them. . . . I really can't be home anymore because of the constant emotional abuse. . . . However, I don't know what to do. I've never asked you for anything, but I am asking you for your advice and support in any way possible. . . . I don't know what to do. I'm falling into a huge depression. . . . What do you think? What should I do?

My worries increase, and I start imagining all the terrible scenarios he might be living. I become angry and sad about my brother and his wife. I go to bed wondering what I am going to say to him when we talk. "What's my role here? Should I ask him how certain he is about his sexual orientation? Is he going to ask me for shelter and, or, money? What and how much should I offer? Should I intercede on his behalf for him with my brother? If I do, how much?" Suddenly, I realize the irony. I have worked all my adult life on LGBT matters. I have worked with, met, and counseled a few hundred gay men. I am finishing a book on the lives of gay men. And yet, here I am, nervous, anxious, and unsure about how to proceed.

I feel some guilt. "This is my own nephew—how could I, how could we, the family, allow this to happen? Why does he have to go through what he calls 'hell'?" I wonder if I should have been more direct and open about my own life with my brothers. I have never talked directly to them about my gay life. My mother and my sister are the only ones in the immediate family with whom I have shared my gay life. My brothers are much older than I. They took care of my sister and me when we were children, when my mother could not afford a *sirvienta* or a *señora* (maid) to look after us. I looked up to them as I was growing up. To a large degree, they were my father figures. They know I am gay and they even have met some of my gay friends and boyfriends. But we have never had an explicit conversation about my sexual orientation or my love life. I love, respect, and support them, and I have always assumed they have the same feelings toward me. But, as my nephew points out about his father, they are rather emotionally reserved. They get angry and sad but rarely talk about their feelings. Our intimacy, thus, is limited.

I wonder if my brother, my nephew's father, is blaming me. I wonder if he is angry with me now that he knows his son is gay. I have not heard from my brother in quite some time. He does not reply to the family emails that every once in a while we, my brothers and sister, exchange. The concern that my brother might blame me first crossed my mind when my nephew visited me three years ago. I invited him to check out several colleges. Since he was in high school, I have encouraged him to move away from El Paso, become independent of his parents, and allow himself to have a wider range of educational and career experiences. We spent a week together, and he met my then-boyfriend. I did not ask about his sexuality. During that time, I wondered if my brother was comfortable having his son stay with me and with my attempts to convince him to go to a college outside of El Paso.

I call my nephew on his cell phone the next day. Without preamble, he begins relating what has happened over the last year or so. His sister found out he had been visiting gay-related websites and told their parents. He acknowledged that he was gay, and his parents told him they would never accept that; the verbal abuse began. He had been asked to move out several times.

As we talk, I hear noises in the background. He is not by himself, and he is getting into a car. It turns out he and his boyfriend are leaving the boyfriend's apartment. They have been together for three months, and my nephew tells me that he is considering moving in with his boyfriend to escape the "emotional abuse" at home. The boyfriend is a few years older and has a better job than my nephew. I sense they are in love. My nephew continues relating the plans they have created. They want to live together and go to school together in another city, far away from El Paso.

I realize I am feeling some envy as he recounts how they met and how they are thinking about the future. It is a strange sensation in my chest. I have been single (and, I believe, happy) for some time. I have fallen in love a few times and pursued two long-term relationships. I have seen love slowly fade through the routine of ordinary life. When I was my nephew's age, I was not in love; I had not fallen in love. I did know I was gay, but I did not have a gay uncle. I was finishing college and being the best student I could be. I was enjoying the experience of learning and discussing social problems and philosophical dilemmas. I was already on my own, miles away from my family. I had begun plotting my future. It was a future in academia. Love and romance seemed too messy and too unpredictable for me to plot and chase. But AIDS, Marco, Oscar, José, and other *compañeros* were on the horizon.

My nephew just wants to talk to me. He needs to talk with someone other than his boyfriend. Before ending our phone conversation, I remind him that he is not alone. He has his (extended) family, and he has me.

APPENDIX

Demographic Information for the Sample of Latino Gay, Bisexual, and Transgender Activists and Volunteers by City, 2001–2002

Characteristics	Chicago n (%) Total n = 40	San Francisco n (%) Total n = 40	Total n (%) Total n = 80
Age			
<29	8 (20)	9 (23)	17 (21)
30–39	23 (57)	16 (40)	39 (49)
40–49	6 (15)	11 (27)	17 (21)
50>	3 (8)	4 (10)	7 (9)
Birthplace			
USA	15 (38)	17 (42)	32 (40)
Mexico	15 (38)	16 (40)	31 (39)
Puerto Rico	5 (13)	1 (3)	6 (7)
Other	5 (13)	6 (15)	11 (14)
Ethnicity if born in the U.S. (n = 32)			
Mexican	9 (60)	14 (82)	23 (72)
Puerto Rican	3 (20)	2 (12)	5 (16)
Other	3 (20)	1 (6)	4 (12)
Education			
Less than high school	5 (13)	4 (10)	9 (11)
High school diploma	2 (5)	4 (10)	6 (8)
Vocational/some college	11 (28)	17 (43)	28 (35)
College graduate	16 (40)	8 (20)	24 (30)
Graduate school	6 (15)	7 (18)	13 (16)
Employment			
Full-time	27 (68)	17 (43)	44 (55)
Part-time	7 (18)	3 (8)	10 (13)
Unemployed	6 (15)	9 (23)	15 (19)
Public aid	0	8 (20)	8 (10)
Student	0	3 (8)	3 (4)
HIV status			
Positive	15 (37)	18 (45)	33 (41)
Negative	23 (57)	22 (55)	45 (56)

REFERENCES

Allahyari, Rebecca A. 2000. *Visions of charity: Volunteer workers and moral community.* Berkeley: University of California Press.

Anthias, Floya. 1990. "Race and class revisited—conceptualizing race and racisms." *Sociological Review* 38:19–42.

Atkinson, Robert. 1998. *The life story interview.* Thousand Oaks, Calif.: Sage Publications.

Bebbington, Andrew C., and Philip N. Gatter. 1994. "Volunteers in an HIV social care organization." *AIDS Care* 6(5): 571–85.

Bellah, Robert N., Richard Madsen, et al. 1996. *Habits of the heart: Individualism and commitment in American life.* Berkeley: University of California Press.

Boehmer, Ulrike. 2000. *The personal and the political: Women's activism in response to the breast cancer and AIDS epidemics.* Albany: State University of New York Press.

Brooks, Ronald, Mary Jane Rotheram-Borus, et al. 2003. "HIV and AIDS among men of color who have sex with men and men of color who have sex with men and women: An epidemiological profile." *AIDS Education and Prevention* 15(1 Suppl A): 1–6.

Brown, Phil, and Edwin J. Mikkelsen. 1990. *No safe place: Toxic waste, leukemia and community action.* Berkeley: University of California Press.

Cable, Sherry. 1992. "Women's social movement involvement: The role of structural availability in recruitment and participation process." *Sociological Quarterly* 33(1): 35–50.

Carrier, Joseph. 1995. *De los otros.* New York: Columbia University Press.

Carrillo, Hector. 2002. *The night is young: Sexuality in Mexico in the times of AIDS.* Chicago: University of Chicago Press.

Catania, Joseph A., Dennis Osmond, et al. 2001. "The continuing HIV epidemic among men who have sex with men." *American Journal of Public Health* 91(6): 907–14.

Centers for Disease Control and Prevention (CDC). 2006. "Racial/ethnic disparities in diagnoses of HIV/AIDS—33 states, 2001–2004." *Morbidity and Mortality Weekly Report (MMWR)* 55(5): 121–25.

Chambré, Susan M. 1991. "Volunteers as witnesses: The mobilization of AIDS volunteers in New York City, 1981–1988." *Social Services Review* 65:531–47.

Chambré, Susan M. 2006. *Fighting for our lives: New York's AIDS community and the politics of disease.* New Brunswick, N.J.: Rutgers University Press.

Chauncey, George. 1994. *Gay New York: Gender, urban culture, and the making of the gay male world, 1890–1940.* New York: Basic Books.

Chodorow, Nancy. 1978. *The reproduction of mothering: Psychoanalysis and the sociology of gender.* Berkeley: University of California Press.

Cochran, Susan D., and Vickie M. Mays. 2000. "Lifetime prevalence of suicide symptoms and affective disorders among men reporting same-sex sexual partners: Results from NHANES III." *American Journal of Public Health* 90(4): 573–78.

Cohen, Cathy J. 1999. *The boundaries of blackness: AIDS and the breakdown of black politics.* Chicago: University of Chicago Press.

Cohen, Sheldon. 1988. "Psychosocial models of the role of social support in the etiology of physical disease." *Health Psychology* 7(3): 269–97.

Cooper, Richard, and Richard David. 1986. "The biological concept of race and its application to epidemiology." *Journal of Health Politics, Policy and Law* 11:97–116.

Cortazzi, Martin. 1993. *Narrative analysis.* London: Falmer Press.

Crimp, Douglas. 2002. *Melancholia and moralism: Essays on AIDS and queer politics.* Cambridge, Mass.: MIT Press.

de Lauretis, Teresa. 1987. *Technologies of gender: Essays on theory, film, and fiction.* Bloomington: Indiana University Press.

Denzin, Norman. 1989. *Interpretive biography.* Newbury Park, Calif.: Sage.

Díaz, Rafael M. 1998. *Latino gay men and HIV: Culture, sexuality, and risk behavior.* New York: Routledge.

Díaz, Rafael M., and George Ayala. 2001. *Social discrimination and health: The case of Latino gay men and HIV risk.* Washington, D.C.: Policy Institute of the National Gay and Lesbian Task Force.

Durkheim, Émile. 1951. *Suicide.* New York: Free Press.

Elliot, Gregory C., Suzanne Kao, and Ann-Marie Grant. 2004. "Mattering: Empirical validation of a social-psychological concept." *Self and Identity* 3:339–54.

Ensel, W. M., and N. Lin. 1991. "The life stress paradigm and psychological distress." *Journal of Health and Social Behavior* 32:321–41.

Epstein, Steven. 1996. *Impure science: AIDS, activism, and the politics of knowledge.* Berkeley: University of California Press.

Eribon, Didier. 2004. *Insult and the making of the gay self.* Durham, N.C.: Duke University Press.

Ewick, Patricia, and Susan Selby. 1995. "Subversive stories and hegemonic tales: Toward a sociology of narrative." *Law and Society Review* 29:197–226.

Feinstein, Jonathan S. 1993. "The relationship between socioeconomic status and health: A review of the literature." *Milbank Quarterly* 71:279–322.

Fife, Betsy, and Eric Wright. 2000. "The dimensionality of stigma: A comparison of its impact on the self of persons with HIV/AIDS and cancer." *Journal of Health and Social Behavior* 41:50–67.

Fisher, Robert. 2005. *Social action community organization: Proliferation, persistence, roots and prospects.* New Brunswick, N.J.: Rutgers University Press.

Foucault, Michel. 1976/1990. *The history of sexuality: An introduction.* New York: Vintage Books.

Frable, Deborrah E., Camille Wortman, et al. 1997. "Predicting self-esteem, well-being, and distress in a cohort of gay men: The importance of cultural stigma, personal visibility, community networks, and positive identity." *Journal of Personality* 65(3): 599–624.

Franke, Katherine M. 2006. "The politics of same sex marriage politics." *Columbia Journal of Gender and Law* 15(1): 237–48.

Fraser, Nancy. 1989. *Unruly practices: Power, discourse, and gender in contemporary social theory.* Minneapolis: University of Minnesota Press.

Freire, Paulo. 1971. *Pedagogy of the oppressed.* New York: Continuum.

Gergen, Mary M. 1988. "Narrative structures and social explanation." In *Analyzing every day explanation: A case of methods,* ed. C. Antaki. London: Sage, 94–112.

Goffman, Erving. 1963. *Stigma: Notes on the management of spoiled identity.* Englewood Cliffs, N.J.: Prentice-Hall.

Gould, Deborah B. 2009. *Moving politics: Emotion and ACT UP's fight against AIDS.* Chicago: University of Chicago Press.

Harris, Daniel. 1997. *The rise and fall of gay culture.* New York: Ballantine.

Hawkins, Ann H. 1990. "A change of heart: The paradigm of regeneration in medical and religious narrative." *Perspectives in Biology and Medicine* 33:547–59.

Heatherton, Todd F., and Patricia A. Nichols. 1994. "Personal accounts of successful versus failed attempts at life change." *Personality and Social Psychology Bulletin* 20(6): 664–75.

Herek, Gregory M. 1999. "AIDS and stigma." *American Behavioral Scientist* 42(7): 1102–12.

House, James S. 1981. *Work, stress, and social support.* Reading, Mass.: Addison-Wesley.

Huebner, David M., M. C. Davis, et al. 2002. "The impact of internalized homophobia on HIV preventive interventions." *American Journal of Community Psychology* 30(3): 327–48.

Hunt, Scott A., Robert Benford, and David Snow. 1994. "Identity fields: Framing process and the social construction of movement identities." In *New social movements: From ideology to identity,* ed. Enrique Larana, Hunk Johnston, and Joseph Gusfield. Philadelphia: Temple University Press, 185–208.

Hydén, Lars-Christer. 1997. "Illness and narrative." *Sociology of Health and Illness* 19(1): 48–69.

Josephson, Jyl. 2005. "Citizenship, same-sex marriage, and feminist critiques of marriage." *Perspectives on Politics* 3(2): 269–84.

Kaiser Family Foundation. 2001. *Inside-OUT: A report on the experiences of lesbians, gays and bisexuals in America and the public's views on issues and policies related to sexual orientation.* Meno Park, Calif.: Kaiser Family Foundation.

Kobasa, Susan C. Ouellette. 1990. "AIDS and volunteer associations: Perspectives on social and individual change." *Milbank Quarterly* 68(S2): 280–94.

Kobasa, Susan C. Ouellette. 1991. "AIDS volunteering: Links to the past and future prospects." In *A disease of society: Cultural and institutional responses to AIDS,* ed. D. Nelkin, D. Willis, and S. Parris. Cambridge: Cambridge University Press, 172–88.

Liberatos, Penny, Bruce G. Link, and J. L. Kelsey. 1988. "The measurement of social class in epidemiology." *Epidemiological Review* 10:87–121.

Link, Bruce G., Elmer L. Struening, et al. 1997. "On stigma and its consequences: Evidence from a longitudinal study of men with dual diagnoses of mental illness and substance abuse." *Journal of Health and Social Behavior* 38(2): 177–90.

Link, Bruce G., and Jo C. Phelan. 2001. "Conceptualizing stigma." *Annual Review of Sociology* 27(1): 363–85.

Loftus, Jeni. 2001. "America's liberalization in attitudes toward homosexuality, 1973 to 1998." *American Sociological Review* 66(5): 762–82.

MacKellar, Duncan A., L. A. Valleroy, et al. 2005. "Unrecognized HIV infection, risk behaviors, and perceptions of risk among young men who have sex with men: Opportunities for advancing HIV prevention in the third decade of HIV/AIDS." *Journal of Acquired Immune Deficiency Syndromes: JAIDS* 38(5): 603–14.

Maines, David. 1993. "Narrative's movement and sociology's phenomena: Toward a narrative sociology." *Sociological Quarterly* 34:17–38.

Martínez, Tomás E. 1995. *Santa Evita.* New York: Vintage Español.

Mason-Schrock, Douglas. 1996. "Transsexuals' narrative construction of the 'true self.'" *Social Psychology Quarterly* 59(3): 176–92.

Mays, Vickie M., and Susan D. Cochran. 2001. "Mental health correlates of perceived discrimination among lesbian, gay and bisexual adults in the United States." *American Journal of Public Health* 91(11): 1869–76.

McAdam, Doug. 1989. "The biographical consequences of activism." *American Sociological Review* 54(5): 744–60.

McDonough, Peggy, and Pat Berglund. 2003. "Histories of poverty and self-rated health trajectories." *Journal of Health and Social Behavior* 33(2): 198–214.

Meyer, Ilan H. 1995. "Minority stress and mental health in gay men." *Journal of Health and Social Behavior* 36:38–56.

Moen, Phyllis, and S. Fields. 1999. *Retirement and well-being: Does community participation replace paid work?* Chicago: American Sociological Association.

Musick, Marc A., and John Wilson. 2008. *Volunteers: A social profile.* Bloomington: Indiana University Press.

Needle, Richard H., Robert T. Trotter II, et al. 2003. "Rapid assessment of the HIV/AIDS crisis in racial and ethnic minority communities: An approach for timely community interventions." *American Journal of Public Health* 93(6): 970–79.

Omoto, Allen M., and A. Lauren Crain. 1995. "AIDS volunteerism: Lesbian and gay community-based responses to HIV." In *AIDS, identity, and community: The HIV epidemic and lesbians and gay men*, ed. G. M. Herek and B. Greene. Thousand Oaks, Calif.: Sage Publications, 187–209.

Parker, Richard G. 1991. *Bodies, pleasure, and passions: Sexual culture in contemporary Brazil*. Boston: Beacon.

Patton, Cindy. 1989. "The AIDS industry: Construction of 'victims,' 'volunteers,' and 'experts.'" In *Taking liberties, AIDS and cultural politics*, ed. E. Carter and S. Watney. London: Serpent's Tail: 113–26.

Paul, Jay P., Joseph Catania, et al. 2002. "Suicide attempts among gay and bisexual men: Lifetime prevalence and antecedents." *American Journal of Public Health* 92(8): 1338–45.

Paz, Octavio. 1962. *The labyrinth of solitude: Life and thought in Mexico*. Translated by Lysander Kemp. New York: Grove Press.

Pearlin, Leonard I., Elizabeth G. Menaghan, et al. 1981. "The stress process." *Journal of Health and Social Behavior* 22(4): 337–56.

Pew Hispanic Center/Kaiser Family Foundation. 2003. *2002 National Survey of Latinos*. Washington, D.C.: Pew Hispanic Center and Kaiser Family Foundation.

Prieur, Annick. 1998. *Mema's house, Mexico City: On transvestites, queens, and machos*. Chicago: University of Chicago Press.

Putnam, Robert D. 2000. *Bowling alone: The collapse and revival of American community*. New York: Simon and Schuster.

Ramirez-Valles, Jesus. 1999. "Changing women: The narrative construction of personal change through community health work among women in Mexico." *Health Education and Behavior* 26(1): 23–40.

Ramirez-Valles, Jesus. 2002. "The protective effects of community involvement for HIV risk behavior: A conceptual framework." *Health Education Research* 17(4): 389–403.

Ramirez-Valles, Jesus, and Amanda U. Brown. 2003. "Latino's community involvement in HIV/AIDS: Organizational and individual perspectives on volunteering." *AIDS Education and Prevention* 15(1 Suppl A): 90–104.

Ramirez-Valles, Jesus, and Rafael M. Díaz. 2005. "Public health, race, and the AIDS movement: The profile and consequences of Latino gay men's community involvement." In *Processes of community change and social action*, ed. A. M. Omoto. Mahwah, N.J.: Lawrence Erlbaum Associates: 51–66.

Ramirez-Valles, Jesus, Stevenson Fergus, et al. 2005. "Confronting stigma: Community involvement and psychological well-being among HIV-positive Latino gay men." *Hispanic Journal of Behavioral Sciences* 27(1): 101–19.

Riessman, Catherine Kohler. 1993. *Narrative analysis*. Newbury Park, Calif.: Sage.

Roediger, David R. 1991. *The wages of whiteness: Race and the making of the American working class*. London: Verso.

Sawicki, Jana. 1991. *Disciplining Foucault: Feminism, power, and the body*. New York: Routledge.

Schieman, Scott, and Joan Taylor. 2001. "Statuses, roles, and the sense of mattering." *Sociological Perspectives* 44:469–84.

Scott, Joan. 1986. "Gender: A useful category of historical analysis." *American Historical Review* 91(5): 1053–75.

Shaw, Randy. 1996. *The activist's handbook: A primer for the 1990s and beyond.* Berkeley: University of California Press.

Sills, David L. 1957. *The volunteers: Means and ends in a national organization.* Glencoe, Ill.: Free Press.

Simon, Bernd, Stefan Stürmer, and Kerstin Steffens. 2000. "Helping individuals or group members? The role of individual and collective identification in AIDS volunteerism." *Personality and Social Psychology Bulletin* 26(4): 497–506.

Skerry, Peter. 1993. *Mexican Americans: Ambivalent minority.* Cambridge, Mass.: Harvard University Press.

Snow, David A., Louis A. Zurcher, and Sheldon Ekland-Olson. 1980. "Social networks and social movements: A microstructural approach to differential recruitment." *American Sociological Review* 45(5): 787–801.

Snow, David A., E. Burke Rochford, Steven K. Worden, and Robert Benford. 1986. "Frame alignment processes, micromobilization, and movement participation." *American Sociological Review* 51(4): 464–81.

Snyder, Mark, and Allen M. Omoto. 1992. "Who helps and why? The psychology of AIDS volunteerism." In *Helping and being helped: Naturalistic studies*, ed. S. Spacapan and S. Oskamp. Newbury Park, Calif.: Sage, 213–39.

Somers, Margaret R. 1992. "Special section: Narrative analysis in social sciences, Part 2. Narrativity, narrative identity, and social action: Rethinking English working class formation." *Social Science History* 16(4): 591–630.

Stockdill, Brett C. 2003. *Activism against AIDS: At the intersections of sexuality, race, gender, and class.* Boulder, Colo.: Lynne Rienner Publishers.

Strub, Sean. 2005. "Fight back, fight AIDS." *Windy City Times.* Chicago, Dec. 28, p. 12.

Tocqueville, Alexis de. 1830/2000. *Democracy in America.* Chicago: University of Chicago Press.

Travisano, Richard V. 1981. "Alternation and conversion as qualitatively different transformations." In *Social psychology through symbolic interaction*, ed. G. Stone. Waltham, Mass.: Ginn-Blaisdell, 594–606.

Turner, Heather A., Robert B. Hays, et al. 1993. "Determinants of social support among gay men: The context of AIDS." *Journal of Health and Social Behavior* 34(1): 37–53.

Varner, Greg. 2005. "Arthur Dong: Lens on homophobic America." *Gay and Lesbian Review* 12:30–31.

Weitz, Rose. 1991. *Life with AIDS.* New Brunswick, N.J.: Rutgers University Press.

Wilkinson, Doris, and Gary King. 1987. "Conceptual and methodological issues in the use of race as a variable: Policy implications." *Milbank Quarterly* 65(S1): 56–71.

Williams, David. R., Harold W. Neighbors, et al. 2003. "Racial/ethnic discrimination and health: Findings from community studies." *American Journal of Public Health* 93(2): 200–208.

Williamson, Ian R. 2000. "Internalized homophobia and health issues affecting lesbians and gay men." *Health Education Research* 15(1): 97–107.

Wolitski, Richard J., Ronald O. Valdiserri, et al. 2001. "Are we headed for a resurgence of the HIV epidemic among men who have sex with men?" *American Journal of Public Health* 91(6): 883–88.

Wolpe, Harold. 1986. "Class concepts, class struggle, and racism." In *Theories of race and ethnic relations,* ed. J. Rex and D. S. Mason. Cambridge: Cambridge University Press, 110–30.

Wright, Erik O., Cynthia Costello, David Hachen, and Joey Sprague. 1982. "The American class structure." *American Sociological Review* 47(6):706–26.

Youniss, James, and Miranda Yates. 1997. *Community service and social responsibility in youth.* Chicago: University of Chicago Press.

INDEX

access to social services and treatment, 127–29, 158–59
activists: actualization of the self in, 152–55; coming out to family, 89–94; *compañeros* as, 79–80, 121–24, 160–61; confidence in, 150–51; critical consciousness and, 151–52; current state of gay, 158; development of the self and, 147–52; growth of gay, 120–21; HIV/AIDS, 3, 104–11, 117–24; importance of, 138–41; media and, 129–31; paid, 133–35; partners and boyfriends of, 135; recruitment of, 124–26; religion and, 135–37, 153; in schools and universities, 131–33; social networks of, 124–27; volunteerism and, 8, 10, 121, 124–27
actualization of the self, 152–55
AIDS Coalition to Unleash Power (ACT UP), 4, 11, 93, 131, 133, 160
AIDS hotlines, 128–29
AIDS Walks, 124, 144
alcoholism, 26, 28
Allahyari, Rebecca A., 8
ALMA (Association of Latino Men for Action), 129–30, 133
Almodóvar, Pedro, 13
Anthias, Floya, 20, 64
Atkinson, Robert, 13
avoidance, 61
Ayala, George, 19, 39

Bebbington, Andrew C., 7
Bellah, Robert N., 7, 10, 11
Beltrán, Lola, 37, 95, 97

Berglund, Pat, 19
bilingual education, 67–68
Boehmer, Ulrike, 7
Brokeback Mountain, 2, 161, 162
Brooks, Ronald, 101
Brown, Amanda U., 8, 137
Brown, Phil, 136
buenas conciencias, Las (Fuentes), 89

Cable, Sherry, 121
candidiasis, 102
Carrier, Joseph, 46
Carrillo, Hector, 39, 46, 94
Castro, Fidel, 10
Catania, Joseph A., 6
Catholicism, 4, 54–55
Centers for Disease Control, 101, 150, 158, 159
Chambré, Susan M., 4, 7, 11
Chauncey, George, 53, 81
children: bilingual education and, 67–68; family influence on, 39–44; of HIV/AIDS patients, 102–3, 109; school and classroom experiences of, 44–47; sexual experiences of, 40, 44, 46, 95–96
civil war, 30, 35–36
Cochran, Susan D., 38, 39
Cohen, Cathy, 8
Cohen, Sheldon, 8
colleges and universities, activism in, 131–33
colonias, 1, 26
coming out to family, 89–94, 161–64
compañeros, 1, 2, 3, 4, 7, 8–11; accessing

services, 127–29; activism by, 79–80, 121–24; on being born gay, 82–84; birth families of, 3–4; children of, 102–3; on entering gay life, 84–89; facing stigma, 60–62; finding Latinoness, 73–76; importance of, 138–39, 164; impoverished, 22–26, 78; "I" *versus* "We" and, 10–11; leadership among, 153–55; life histories of, 13–17; marriages to women, 87–89; media and, 129–31; middle class, 31–35; negative consequences of stigma for, 57–59; racism experienced by, 66–71; rebellion and, 81; recruitment of, 124–27; segregation of, 71–72; self-acceptance by, 139–40; the self and, 7–11, 145–52; self-identification by, 4–5, 141–44; sense of community among, 8; social-class origins of, 21–22; solidarity and ideology among, 157–58, 160–61; supporting those with HIV/AIDS, 104–11; transgender, 94–99; wealthy, 35–36, 58; and the white AIDS movement in the U.S., 6–7; working class, 27–31
confidence, 150–51
consciousness: creation of, 76–80; critical, 151–52
Cooper, Richard, 11, 64
Cortazzi, Martin, 14
Crain, A. Lauren, 7
creation of consciousness, 76–80
Crimp, Douglas, 6, 158, 159
critical consciousness, 151–52
cross dressing, 37–38, 40, 95–96, 145; police harassment and, 50–51
culture, Latino, 75–76

David, Richard, 11, 64
de Lauretis, Teresa, 81
Denzin, Norman, 13, 140, 141
diagnoses of HIV/AIDS, 101–4
Díaz, Rafael M., 8, 19, 39, 46, 92
dislocation, 51–53
Dong, Arthur, 158
"don't-ask-don't-tell" attitude, 61
drug abuse, 29, 35
Durkheim, Émile, 8

eating disorders, 54
education, bilingual, 67–68

Elliot, Gregory C., 153
En La Vida, 129, 130
Ensel, W. M., 8, 60
Epstein, Steven, 4
Eribon, Didier, 160, 161
Ewick, Patricia, 14, 81

"fallo positivo," 101–4
family: activism and, 124–27; coming out to, 89–94, 161–64; concept of, 12; influence on gender conformity, 39–44; support of HIV/AIDS patients, 104–11
farm workers, 23–25
fathers, stigmatization of gay sons by, 41–42
Feinstein, Jonathan S., 19
Félix, María, 13
Fields, S., 8
Fife, Betsy, 38
Fisher, Robert, 4
Foucault, Michel, 63, 81
Frable, Deborrah E., 8, 39
Franke, Katherine M., 159
Fraser, Nancy, 64
Freire, Paulo, 64, 68, 76, 151
Fuentes, Carlos, 89

Gatter, Philip N., 7
Gay, Lesbian and Bisexual Veterans, 133
Gay, Lesbian and Straight Education Network, 132
Gay Chicago, 129
gender nonconformity: dislocation due to, 51–53; family influence and, 39–44; internalization and, 53–57, 78–79; negative consequences of the stigma associated with, 57–62; police harassment due to, 49–51; school and classroom experiences affecting, 44–47; stigma toward, 38–39; therapy and, 47–49
Gergen, Mary M., 14
Goffman, Erving, 38
Gould, Deborah, 10, 11
guilt, 84

Habits of the Heart, 10
harassment: police, 49–51; sexual, 47
Harris, Daniel, 158
Hawkins, Ann H., 140

Heatherton, Todd F., 141
histories, life, 13–17
HIV/AIDS: access to services for, 127–29;
    activism in schools and universities,
    131–33; books on, 92–93; changing
    the self, 111–16; children of men with,
    102–3, 109; commercialization of, 5–6;
    current state of activism and services for,
    158–59; diagnosis of, 101–4; education
    programs, 119; "fallo positivo" and,
    101–4; initial appearance of, 1, 158; me-
    dia and, 129–31; melancholy and, 6; paid
    activists, 133–35; prevention and services
    among Latinos and, 1–2; support of fam-
    ily, boyfriends, and *compañeros* for those
    with, 104–11; volunteer recruitment and,
    124–27. *See also* activists
hormone therapy, 97–98
hotlines, AIDS, 128–29
House, James S., 8
Huebner, David M., 39
Hunt, Scott A., 121
Hydén Lars-Christer, 14

immigration, 11–12; dislocation and,
    51–53; poverty and, 22–23
insults, 69, 73
internalization, 53–57, 78–79
"I" *versus* "We," 10–11

Jehovah's Witnesses, 52–53, 58
Josephson, Jyl, 159

Kaiser Foundation, 7, 39
King, Gary, 11, 64
Kobasa, Susan C. Ouellette, 4, 7, 8

Latinoness, 11–13, 73–76
Latinos: as a category, 63; creation of
    consciousness by, 76–80; identity, 64–66,
    141–44; and Latinoness, 11–13, 73–76;
    as a minority group, 64; race and, 63–64
leadership, 153–55
Lee, Ang, 2
Liberatos, Penny, 20
life histories, 13–17
Lin, N., 8, 60
Link, Bruce G., 38
Loftus, Jeni, 39

machismo, 41–42, 60
MacKellar, Duncan A., 101
Making Love, 162
mannerisms, 44, 46, 52
maquiladoras, 2
María Victoria, 95
marriage, 87–89, 159
Martínez, Tomás E., 1
Masson-Shrock, Douglas, 94
Mays, Vickie M., 38, 39
McAdam, Doug, 115, 140, 141
McDonough, Peggy, 19
media, 129–31
melancholy, 6
Meyer, Ilan H., 8, 38, 39, 60
middle class, the, 31–35
Mikkelsen, Edwin J., 136
misogyny, 57
mockery, 45–47
Moen, Phyllis, 8
morenos, 73
mothers: concept of, 13; of HIV/AIDS pa-
    tients, 105–6, 109; stigmatization of gay
    sons by, 42–43
Moving Politics, 10
Musick, Marc A., 9

name-calling, 45–46
National Institutes of Health, 4, 159
Needle, Richard H., 101
negative consequences of stigma, 57–59
Nichols, Patricia A., 141
Norte, El, 1

objectification, 69–70
Omoto, Allen M., 7

paid activists, 133–35
paisanos, 133–34
Parker, Richard G., 46
Patton, Cindy, 5
Paz, Octavio, 13, 74
Pearlin, Leonard I., 8, 60
Perón, Eva, 13
Pew Hispanic Center, 7
Phelan, Jo C., 38, 39
physical abuse, 44, 47; by police, 50
police harassment, 49–51
poor, the, 22–26, 78

Poz magazine, 5–6
Prieur, Annick, 46
psychotherapy, 47–49, 87
public housing, 29
Putnam, Robert D., 10

Queer Nation, 133

race, concept of, 63–64
racism, 11, 26; among white gays, 71–72;
    bilingual education and, 67–68; experi-
    enced by *compañeros*, 66–71; objectifica-
    tion as, 69–70; rejection and, 68–69; skin
    color and, 72–73
Ramirez-Valles, Jesus, 8, 19, 38, 56, 115,
    137, 140; activism, 118–20; on the com-
    ing out process, 161–64; departure from
    Mexico, 156–57; early work on HIV/
    AIDS, 1–6; family of, 161–64; life histo-
    ries collected by, 14–15; social-class and,
    19–20; study interests of, 6–7
rebellion, 81
recruitment of activists, 124–27
rejection as stigma, 68–69
religion: activism and, 135–37, 153; gender
    expectations and, 4, 52–53, 54–55, 58,
    60–61
ridicule, 45–47
Riessman, Catherine Kohler, 13
Roediger, David R., 20, 64

Sawicki, Jana, 81
Schieman, Scott, 153
school and classroom experiences: activism
    and, 131–33; of children, 44–47
Scott, Joan, 81
segregation in gay communities, 71–72
Selby, Susan, 14, 81
self: activism and the, 7–8; actualization
    of the, 152–55; development of the,
    149–52; development of the gay and
    transgender, 145–47; development of the
    HIV-positive and sexual, 147–49; HIV/
    AIDS changing the, 111–16, 147–49
self-acceptance, 84–89; as *compañeros*,
    139–40
self-identification, 4–5, 8; after marriages,
    87–89; becoming a gay man and, 82–94;

coming out to family and, 89–94; in the
    company of others, 99; internalization
    of stigma and, 53–57; as a Latino gay
    man, 141–44; by Latinos, 64–66; self-
    acceptance and, 84–89; transgenders and,
    94–99
Sentinel, 130
sexual experiences of children, 40, 44, 46,
    95–96
sexual harassment, 47
sex workers, 1–2
Shanti, 139, 140
Shaw, Randy, 4
Sills, David, 136
Simon, Bernd, 121
Skerry, Peter, 63, 64
skin color, 72–73
Snow, David, 121
Snyder, Mark, 7
social-class origins, 19–22; assessment of,
    21; of *compañeros*, 20–22; and deter-
    mination of class position, 20–21; im-
    poverished, 22–26; middle class, 31–35;
    skin color and, 72–73; wealthy, 35–36;
    working class, 27–31
social networks, 124–27
social services access, 127–29
solidarity and ideology among *compañeros*,
    157–58, 160–61
Somers, Margaret R., 14
stigma, 38–39; coming out and, 90–91;
    dislocation and, 51–53; facing, 60–62; by
    family, 40–44; internalization of, 53–57,
    78–79; negative consequences of, 57–59;
    racism and, 66–71; rejection as, 68–69;
    by school children, 45–46
Stockdill, Brett C., 11
St. Patrick's Roman Catholic Cathedral, 4
Strub, Sean, 5–6
substance abuse, 29, 35
suicide, 59, 102
support groups, 107–8. *See also* activists

Taylor, Joan, 153
therapy, 47–49, 87; hormone, 97–98
Tocqueville, Alexis de, 10
transgenders, 94–95; cross dressing by,
    37–38, 40, 95–96; police harassment of,

49–51; self, development of the, 145–47; transformation of, 96–99
Travisano, Richard V., 115, 141
treatments, HIV/AIDS, 127–52, 158–59
Turner, Heather A., 8

United Church of Christ, 136

Varner, Greg, 158
Virgin of Guadalupe, the, 13
volunteerism, 8, 10, 121; friends and family involved in, 124–27; importance of, 138–41; the self and, 147–49

war, 30, 35–36
wealthy, the, 35–36, 58
Weitz, Rose, 8
"whitewashed" Latinos, 74, 78
Wilkinson, Doris, 11, 64
Williams, David R., 8
Williamson, Ian R., 39
Wilson, John, 9
Windy City Times, 129
Wolitski, Richard J., 6
Wolpe, Harold, 20, 64
working class, the, 27–31
Wright, Erik O., 20, 38

LATINOS IN CHICAGO AND THE MIDWEST

Pots of Promise: Mexicans and Pottery at Hull-House, 1920–40
  Edited by Cheryl R. Ganz and Margaret Strobel
Moving Beyond Borders: Julian Samora and the Establishment of Latino
  Studies   Edited by Alberto López Pulido, Barbara Driscoll de Alvarado,
  and Carmen Samora
¡Marcha! Latino Chicago and the Immigrant Rights Movement
  Edited by Amalia Pallares and Nilda Flores-González
Bringing Aztlán to Chicago: My Life, My Work, My Art
  José Gamaliel González, edited and with an Introduction
  by Marc Zimmerman
Latino Urban Ethnography and the Work of Elena Padilla
  Edited by Mérida M. Rúa
Defending Their Own in the Cold: The Cultural Turns of U.S.
  Puerto Ricans   Marc Zimmerman
Chicanas of 18th Street: Narratives of a Movement from Latino
  Chicago   Leonard G. Ramírez with Yenelli Flores, María Gamboa,
  Isaura González, Victoria Pérez, Magda Ramírez-Castañeda,
  and Cristina Vital
Compañeros: Latino Activists in the Face of AIDS   Jesus Ramirez-Valles

JESUS RAMIREZ-VALLES is a professor of community health sciences at the University of Illinois, Chicago.

The University of Illinois Press
is a founding member of the
Association of American University Presses.

———————————————————————

Composed in 10/13 Sabon LT Std
by Celia Shapland
at the University of Illinois Press
Manufactured by Thomson-Shore, Inc.

University of Illinois Press
1325 South Oak Street
Champaign, IL 61820-6903
www.press.uillinois.edu